Mental Health Today
a handbook

Edited by Catherine Jackson and Kathryn Hill

Mental Health Today
A handbook

Published by:
Pavilion Publishing (Brighton) Ltd
Richmond House
Richmond Road
Brighton BN2 3RL
Tel: 01273 623222
Fax: 01273 625526
Email: info@pavpub.com
Web: www.pavpub.com

In association with:
The Mental Health Foundation
Sea Containers House
20 Upper Ground
London SE1 9QB

First published 2006. Reprinted 2007.

ISBN-10: 1 84196 171 X
ISBN-13: 978 1 84196 171 2

Pavilion is the leading training and development provider and publisher in the health, social care and allied fields, providing a range of innovative training solutions underpinned by sound research and professional values. We aim to put our customers first, through excellent customer service and good value.

Editors: Catherine Jackson and Kathryn Hill
Cover design: Art Matters
Page layout and typesetting: Faye Thompson
Printing: Ashford Press (Southampton)

Mental Health Today

a handbook

Edited by Catherine Jackson and Kathryn Hill

Contents

Foreword

This book is intended to challenge and inspire all those wishing to develop a stronger vision of what mental health is about, how it can be improved, and what can be done about mental ill health. It is aimed particularly at support workers, at all those providing front-line care in the statutory and voluntary mental health sectors, at service users and carers, and also at generic health workers whose practice would benefit from knowing more about the issues it covers. It is intended to complement the level 2 and 3 certificates in community mental health care, which have allowed many such people to access high quality training and qualifications.

Support workers play a key role in services. Often they are the staff most valued by service users for the practical help they offer that can make so much difference to the quality of people's lives. In the past they have often been left vulnerable and ill-equipped to deal with the issues they encounter, but thankfully this is changing. It is clearer and clearer just how much impact front line staff – whether professionally qualified or not – and people working in other public services – teachers, the police, receptionists – can have on people's lives. That is why we at the Mental Health Foundation and Pavilion believe it is so important to look beyond the traditional mental health professions for impact and change.

It is important that we all grasp the context in which people 'have' mental health or ill health. This context includes policy, society, family life, our biology, our origins as a species, and our collective understanding of mental health and fears about mental ill health. This book attempts to develop our understanding. I have long argued for an 'integrative' approach that looks at medical, social, psychological and experiential, personal perspectives, and values them equally. I explain more in my opening chapter to the book. In order to take that approach to its logical conclusion we will have to offer a much wider range of responses to mental health and ill health and to include people with more serious mental ill health in a range of opportunities. This requires more than just a risk management approach, which is often over-emphasised in government policy.

Often front-line staff have few opportunities to take time out to reflect on these wider perspectives. Yet the emphasis on continuing professional development and lifelong education suggests that more such opportunities should be available. I hope that this book provides such opportunities to the individuals and the organisations in which they work that are committed to personal and service development.

Andrew McCulloch *Chief executive, the Mental Health Foundation*

Contributors

Geoff Brennan is a registered nurse for the mentally handicapped and a registered mental nurse. Geoff has worked in a variety of clinical and academic posts, mainly in London. For four years Geoff also worked with Rethink (then the National Schizophrenia Fellowship) and has practised and taught psychosocial interventions for psychosis since the early 90s. Throughout his career Geoff has maintained an active involvement with acute inpatient care, including working for six years in London services. He carried out the benchmarking of London inpatient services for the Health and Social Care Advisory Service/London Development Centre and was one of two City Nurses working in East London to improve wards. In January 2006 Geoff took up the post of nurse consultant, psychosocial interventions with Berkshire Healthcare NHS Trust. This post, based at Prospect Park Hospital in Reading, has confirmed his admiration for inpatient nurses and the teams they work within.

Tina Coldham has been a user of mental health services for the past 16 years. She has used this experience to become self-employed as a trainer/lecturer, researcher and consultant, promoting user/survivor perspectives in all her work. Tina started working as a community mental health development worker in a voluntary sector project local to her, where she implemented a range of initiatives to help empower fellow users. In 2001 she became a research associate for the Centre for Mental Health Services Development England, Kings College London, where she worked on the three-year national pilot to implement direct payments in mental health. She now works as a national development consultant for the Health and Social Care Advisory Service (HASCAS) and took part in the review Making a Real Difference: strengthening service user and carer involvement in NIMHE. Tina was recently re-elected to the national advisory panel for MindLink, the user/survivor arm of national Mind, and is a member of the Partners Council at the Social Care Institute for Excellence (SCIE). However, Tina still finds time to actively campaign for better mental health services at grass roots level.

Jeanette Copperman has a background in community development and advice work in the voluntary sector and in policy work in local authorities and in the NHS. She has worked with travellers and was a founder member of the National Women and Mental Health Network, a coalition of mental health service users and professionals, and is the women's lead for the Social Perspectives Network based at the Social Care Institute for Excellence. She has interests in and has written about user involvement, women and mental health, gender issues, interprofessional practice and on issues of harassment and abuse. She is currently senior lecturer in social work at City University where she was appointed to foster social work input into the MSc programmes in interprofessional practice, including a programme for practitioners working with survivors of violence. In recent years she has completed research projects with the Kings Fund, the Sainsbury Centre for Mental Health and Barnardos.

David Crepaz-Keay is senior policy advisor on patient and public involvement at the Mental Health Foundation. In this role he undertakes research, develops services, designs training, influences policy and raises public awareness to help people survive, recover from and avoid mental distress. Prior to this he was chief executive of Mental Health Media, an organisation that challenges discrimination and exclusion of people with a psychiatric label. David is a passionate campaigner against discrimination on grounds of mental health history. With over 25 years of involvement, first as a user of mental health services and later as a campaigner, he is also an advocate of service user voices being included in mental health service planning and delivery. David is also a commissioner with the Commission for Patient and Public Involvement in Health, and currently its vice chair.

Janine Fletcher is a mental health nurse currently completing her PhD on case management for depression, funded by the Department of Health. She has visited sites in the US where the treatment of common mental health problems is advanced and subsequently has been involved in developing and evaluating systems of care relevant to the UK. She also works for NIMHE as primary care facilitator and project manager of a collaborative involving the implementation of graduate workers using self-help interventions in a stepped care model of service delivery. She has also written a commissioning guide for primary care based on the implementation of the NICE guideline for depression. Janine is trained in cognitive behaviour therapy and has worked in and managed a number of primary care mental health services. She continues to work closely with primary care and delivers a suicide prevention training package (Skills Based Training on Risk Management (STORM)) for both primary and secondary care services.

Lynne Friedli is editor of the Journal of Public Mental Health and author of Making it Possible: improving mental health and well-being in England, the NIMHE/CSIP public mental health framework. She was founding chief executive of the mental health promotion charity mentality, where she led on the production of the Department of Health guide to mental health promotion, Making it Happen. She left mentality in 2002 to set up her own consultancy and now works across the UK and Europe on the development of public mental health policy and practice.

Fiona Hill has been the director of Brent Mental Health User Group (BUG), an independent user group, for approaching six years and has been involved with the London Development Centre for Mental Health since its beginning. She also works as a trainer and writer on a consultancy basis and has been using mental health services for about 11 years. She has worked in the voluntary sector for more years than she cares to remember and feels she was probably born campaigning. She has worked around lots of issues, particularly in relation to women, lesbians and disabled women, and has been involved with many different kinds of user groups. She has two cats, commonly known as 'the boys', who are a great help, particularly when writing…

Kathryn Hill began working in mental health in 1989 when she commissioned and subsequently managed a psychiatric inpatient unit. Kathryn then went on to be a locality director of mental health services in a large London mental health trust, where she introduced integrated CMHTs and assertive outreach teams. Kathryn has also worked as a service development consultant/research fellow for the Institute for Applied Health and Social Policy, where she led on a number of projects relating to service reconfiguration, whole system working and supporting the implementation of the national service framework for mental health. Kathryn was the mental health lead at the National Patient Safety Agency, where she worked closely with the Department of Health to develop and issue new guidance relating to adverse events in mental health services. She has published widely on this subject. She is currently the director of mental health programmes at the Mental Health Foundation, where she is responsible for policy, research, service improvement, workforce development and patient and public involvement.

Catherine Jackson is editor of the monthly magazine Mental Health Today, published by Pavilion, which she launched in 2001. Previously she edited the mental health nursing journals Mental Health Care and Mental Health Nursing. She has specialised in health journalism for most of her working career, first as a cartoonist for Nursing Times, then a reporter on Nursing Standard, and as deputy editor of the Health Visitor journal for eight years before specialising in mental health issues.

Frank Keating is a senior lecturer in health and social care at Royal Holloway University of London. He was lead author for the Breaking the Circles of Fear report, published by the Sainsbury Centre for Mental Health. This report reviewed the troubled relationship between African and Caribbean communities and mental health services in England. A number of the recommendations of the report have been included in the Department of Health's framework for Delivering Race Equality. Frank is an advisor to a number of organisations on issues of race equality and has recently served on one of the advisory panels of the Disability Rights Commission's formal investigation into health inequalities. Frank continues to publish and conduct research in the field of race equality and mental health.

Sarah Kendal qualified as a mental health nurse in 1991. She has worked in secondary care, primary care and the primary/secondary care interface, mainly in the community in central Manchester. She was instrumental in setting up a primary care service based on guided self-help. She benefited from a clinical scholarship scheme run between Manchester University and the local primary care trusts, and subsequently won a Florence Nightingale Foundation travel award. At present she is a practitioner fellow at Manchester University, developing a guided self-help intervention to promote emotional health in teenagers.

Paul Lelliott is the director of the Royal College of Psychiatrists' research and training unit. In that capacity, he leads a programme of mental health services research and multi-centre quality improvement initiatives. The former includes national studies about the range of mental health residential services. The latter include the Healthcare Commission's national audit of violence in inpatient settings and the new accreditation system for acute psychiatric wards. Details of the unit's work can be found at http://www.rcpsych.ac.uk/crtu.aspx. Dr Lelliott is also a consultant psychiatrist employed by Oxleas NHS Trust. His clinical work is centred on a busy community mental health team in south east London. He is mental health clinical specialty adviser to the National Patient Safety Agency, a member of the Partners Council of the National Institute for Health and Clinical Excellence and a member of the mental health advisory board of the Healthcare Commission.

Ros Levenson is an independent researcher and policy consultant. She has a particular interest in older people and in mental health. She is the joint author of London's State of Mind, the report of an inquiry into mental health in London, published by the King's Fund, and she has written about older people and tackling age discrimination for the King's Fund and the Department of Health. Ros also has a long-term interest in patient and public involvement. She is also a non-executive director of an NHS trust.

Louise Lingwood has over 20 years experience of managing mental health services across health and social care, including inpatient, community and day services. Having originally trained as a social worker, she has also undertaken service reviews and inspections on behalf of the Healthcare Commission. Louise has a particular interest in day services modernisation and is an active member of a national forum for day services development. As a former associate of the London Development Centre for Mental Health she authored the 2005 CSIP publication Redesigning Day Services, a modernisation toolkit for London, as a contribution to the Mental Health and Social Exclusion report implementation in the capital. Louise is currently on secondment from CNWL Mental Health Trust to the Mental Health Foundation, where she is project manager of a Department of Health funded third sector workforce development project.

Liz Main is an independent mental health consultant and journalist. She was a member of the mental health expert task group for the Department of Health's Choice, Equity and Responsiveness consultation in 2002/03. In 2004 she worked for the Social Exclusion Unit in the Department of Health as a policy advisor for the report Mental Health and Social Exclusion. She has advised the government on a variety of mental health policy issues, including tackling stigma and discrimination, and works closely with the voluntary sector, including with the Mental Health Alliance to contest the Mental Health Bill. She has used secondary mental health services in the UK since 1999, including several hospital admissions where she had little choice over not just her treatment, but even the most minor decisions such as when to eat or sleep.

Andrew McCulloch has been chief executive of the Mental Health Foundation for four years. Prior to this appointment he was director of policy at the Sainsbury Centre for Mental Health for six years. He was formerly a civil servant in the Department for Health for 16 years and was responsible for mental health and learning disabilities policy from 1992 to 1996. He has particular interests in policy development, partnership working, models of care, human resources and public mental health. He has spoken and published widely. His other experience has included being a school governor, the non-executive director of an NHS trust (where he was chair of Mental Health Act managers), and chair of Mental Health Media, a charity dedicated to giving a voice to people with mental health problems and learning disabilities.

Andrew Nocon is a senior research officer at the Disability Rights Commission. He has a background in both social work and social and health care research. He has worked in generic social services, taught on a social work course, and carried out research with users of mental health services and on outcomes of community care, the service needs of disabled people, and primary healthcare services. He has worked on ways to ensure that service users are centrally involved in research. Andrew co-ordinated the research input into the Disability Rights Commission's formal investigation into health inequalities experienced by people with mental health problems and/or learning disabilities.

Steve Onyett is senior development consultant for the Care Services Improvement Partnership in the south west (CSIP-SW) and visiting professor at the Faculty of Health and Social Care at the University of the West of England. He has worked as practitioner, service development consultant, manager, trainer and researcher and has published widely, including Teamworking in Mental Health (Palgrave Macmillan, 2003). He moved to the south west in 1998 from south Kent, where he was head of clinical psychology. His previous roles include founding and managing an inner London community mental health team providing assertive community treatment. This experience formed the basis of Case Management in Mental Health (Stanley Thornes, 1998). More recently he has been working with Aston Business School on the Effective Teamworking and Leadership in Mental Health programme, which was rolled out through CSIP development centres. In his current role he leads on issues concerning leadership and teamworking, particularly as they relate to the promotion of social inclusion, and has recently completed a national survey of crisis resolution teams.

Tony Ryan has worked in service and organisational development since 2000, undertaking a wide range of development, evaluation and research initiatives across England and Wales in the fields of mental health, alcohol misuse, substance misuse and learning disabilities. He has completed work for a variety of organisations, including primary care trusts, strategic health authorities, the National Institute for Mental Health in England, the National Patient Safety Agency, specialist mental health providers, local authority social services departments and a number of voluntary and user organisations. Tony also has 10 years clinical experience working in the NHS as a nurse and eight years in the voluntary sector with the national charity Turning Point. He was awarded his PhD from Lancaster University in 2000 and has published on mental health policy, research methods and service and practice development. Tony edited Managing Crisis and Risk for Mental Health Nursing (1999) and co-edited Good Practice in Adult Mental Health (2004) and New Approaches to Suicide Prevention (2004). He is director of Tony Ryan Associates, which was established in December 2004.

Iain Ryrie trained as a mental health nurse in 1983 and has worked both clinically and academically in this field for over 20 years. Iain has been responsible for the development and management of multidisciplinary services in hospital and community settings, and has held positions at King's College, London and at the Sainsbury Centre for Mental Health, where he was head of research before joining the Mental Health Foundation as their research programme director. Iain's published work in the mental health field includes more than 30 peer review articles, chapter contributions to textbooks and commissioned reports for a national audience.

Liz Sayce is director, policy and communications for the Disability Rights Commission, with responsibility for policy development, research, strategy and all aspects of communications. Previously she was director of Lambeth, Southwark and Lewisham Health Action Zone. She spent eight years as policy director of Mind, and one year as a Harkness Fellow in the US, studying the impact of the Americans with Disabilities Act and related policy initiatives. She was a member of the government's Disability Rights Task Force (1997-99). She has published widely on mental health and disability issues and led the Disability Rights Commission's formal investigation into health inequalities experienced by people with mental health problems and/or learning disabilities.

David Seward was until recently director of service development at the Sainsbury Centre for Mental Health and is now one of four directors at Research and Development in Mental Health (RDMH). RDMH has been created to continue mainstream service and workforce development following the change of focus at SCMH to employment and prison mental health. While at SCMH, David contributed to its thinking on the future for commissioning and chaired the conference 'Commissioning Mental Health Services in the New NHS: Tensions and Opportunities'. He has also written a number of articles on commissioning. He previously worked in mental health for over 15 years, holding a number of operational and senior management posts. He has direct experience of commissioning mental health and substance misuse services and has headed up numerous initiatives designed to improve commissioning systems and outcomes. Over the last few years he has specialised in supporting organisational change, with a specific emphasis on facilitating partnership working.

Graham Thornicroft is professor of community psychiatry and head of the multidisciplinary health services research department at the Institute of Psychiatry, King's College London. He is a consultant psychiatrist and director of research and development at the South London and Maudsley NHS Trust. He chaired the external reference group for the national service framework for mental health in England. His areas of research expertise include stigma and discrimination, mental health needs assessment, the development of outcome scales, cost-effectiveness evaluation of mental health treatments, and mental health services in less economically developed countries. He has authored and co-authored 20 books and over 160 papers in peer reviewed journals.

Alan Worthington retired early in 1989 from running a community college science department to provide care to identical twin sons who were encountering mental health problems in adolescence. Fostered from age two years, their journeys have provided many insights into their illness and the responses by services. His experiences as a carer resulted in the appointment in 1991 in the pioneering role of carers support worker to develop and deliver support services for other carers in Exeter. This brought him into contact with a large number of families, and their experiences helped to shape future work. Alan served in this role until 2001 and continues as a carer activist to press the case for co-ordinated and comprehensive responses to carer needs. He also champions decent care for loved ones. Currently he is a member of the NIMHE national acute care steering group and the national acute mental health project board. Locally he chairs the Devon Partnership Trust public patient involvement forum and attends Exeter Relatives Forum.

Introduction

Adult mental health services have been transformed almost beyond recognition in the past 20 years. They have moved from a primarily custodial system, where the majority of patients were warehoused in long-stay institutions, to today's community-based services operating in a policy context that emphasises social inclusion and recovery.

This book can only hope to give a partial picture of a highly complex field: of the breadth of policies that impact on mental health, and the care and treatment of mental ill health; the wealth of good practice, and the debates about the key issues of human rights, treatment models and even what constitutes mental health and ill health. A constant theme throughout is the tension that has always characterised mental health policies and practice: between control of a group of people seen to pose a high risk to themselves and to others, and their right to the self-determination and choice available to all other users of health services. Another key theme is what constitutes effective treatment, and who defines effectiveness. In an arena of healthcare practice that, some argue, lacks a biological basis for the medical interventions that are still the first-line response to a diagnosis.

The book is structured broadly around the seven standards of the national service framework for mental health (Department of Health, 1999), and the review five years into its ten-year implementation (Appleby, 2004). These set out the national priorities for reform and the direction of government policy on adult mental health. It is presented in themes, rather than structured strictly according to the standards, and also includes a chapter on the mental health of older people, which is more usually categorised under the national service framework for older people. We have not attempted to cover children's mental health and services: this is a topic that requires its own, separate volume. Of course, it is impossible to do justice to the mental health needs of older people in a single chapter, but (as the chapter argues) their needs are in many cases no different from those of younger, working age adults; the difference lies more in the inadequacy of health service responses.

The book is also intended to support students taking the level 2 and 3 certificates in community mental health care developed by the Mental Health Foundation with Pavilion. Its aim in this respect is the same as it is for any other reader: to offer a snapshot of the current state of play in a constantly evolving (and revolving) scenario, and of the key debates and how they are being addressed, and to prompt and encourage reflection and further exploration of the topics and challenges it describes.

We start with the fundamental question underpinning mental health policy and practice: how we conceptualise and describe mental health and its corollary, mental ill health. We end with an attempt to show how the process of commissioning mental health services – that is, the mechanisms whereby government funds are translated into services on the ground – is central to the delivery of the government's social inclusion agenda for people with mental health problems. Between these two extremes we attempt to describe the component parts that together create a coherent picture of current national policy and mental health practice, and the key debates that inform them. We cover race and race discrimination; mental health as a continuum and as a public health issue; the mental health needs of women and of older people; service user involvement; choice and user empowerment; mental health in primary care; the crisis in acute services, and the care and treatment of people with the most complex and challenging mental health needs.

We do not specifically address mental health legislation. While the general direction of government policy on this issue is clear, the mechanics of its implementation remained in flux as this book was being prepared.

Inevitably new policies will have emerged in the time it takes to bring a book from manuscript to publication. But we would argue that the broad parameters and the main themes and areas of contention have changed very little over the centuries, and it is these, as well as their current manifestations, with which this book is concerned.

Looking to the future, it is clear that structural changes and reorganisations will continue, as will the debates about funding and resources. The national service framework for mental health is also approaching its tenth anniversary (2010), and it is timely to start thinking now about what should come next. Certainly, as practitioners and services become more recovery-focused, they will need to change both the way they work and the way in which services are delivered so that user-centred care becomes a reality that supports individuals on the recovery journey of their choice. A national service framework for the next decade should be not just about models of service provision. There should be a new way of thinking that embraces a mental health approach, rather than a mental illness approach, and that covers all spectrums and all ages.

Catherine Jackson and Kathryn Hill

References

Appleby L (2004) *The national service framework for mental health – five years on.* London: Department of Health.

Department of Health (1999) *National service framework for mental health: modern standards and service models.* London: Department of Health.

Chapter 1
Understanding mental health and mental illness

Andrew McCulloch

Most people are in a fog about mental health and mental illness and the relationship between the two. Even distinguished professionals and researchers in the mental health sector often propose simplistic models (eg. the single continuum model, from extreme mental ill health to perfect mental health) that defy both the evidence and people's lived experience. But, equally, arrogance must be avoided. No single model can explain a part of human experience so rich as mental health and so threatening and diverse as mental illness. This chapter seeks to explain some of the thinking around models of mental health and ill health and to propose a way forward: an integrative approach, drawing on a range of explanations.

Mental health

While understandings of mental illness go back to ancient times, mental health is essentially a modern concept. Literature from the past explores various mental states, including pure happiness ('Rarely, rarely comest thou,/Spirit of Delight' – Song, by PB Shelley), contentment and functionality. To some extent this reflects current thinking and confusions about mental health. While we argue that mental health does not equate to happiness, this is a common belief in the field of mental health promotion and in other literature (Layard, 2005).

The World Health Organisation's constitution (WHO, 1946) defines health as:

> '… a state of complete physical, mental and social well-being and not merely the absence of disease and infirmity.'

Modern definitions of mental health stem from the idea that there is a state of positive health that is more than just the absence of illness, and that can indeed co-exist with illness. In other words, a mentally healthy person can become depressed under certain circumstances, just as a physically healthy person can acquire an injury or infection.

Mental illness

Mental illness has been recognised since ancient times, when it was attributed to a variety of causes, including demonic possession ('My name is Legion: for we are many' – Mark 5:9, the Bible, King James Version). Over the centuries many models of mental illness have emerged and evolved, which have been summarised by various authors.

Mental illness as a concept has fundamental importance to people's lives, which mental health simply does not. This is because definitional systems of mental illness are used by society to classify, control and treat those thought to be mentally ill. The uses of models of mental illness as part of our social structure mean that there is much more debate about mental illness than there is about mental health.

Understanding mental health

Mental health is a fundamental platform for our existence as human beings. In some ways it is more important than physical health, although inseparable from it. Mental health includes healthy thinking (cognition), emotions (emotional health) and perception (interpreting what our senses tell us, which involves both thinking and feeling). Very poor mental health is something we all fear, and this perhaps tells us how much we value our mental health, even if we do not think much about it.

The Mental Health Foundation defines mental health as follows:

'A state of well-being in which the individual realises his or her own abilities, can cope with the normal stresses of life, can work productively and fruitfully, and is able to make a contribution to his or her community.' (www.mentalhealth.org.uk)

It has also been defined as including:

'… a positive sense of well-being; individual resources including self-esteem, optimism, a sense of mastery and coherence; the ability to initiate, develop and sustain mutually satisfying relationships and the ability to cope with adversities.' (Jenkins et al, 2002)

The important point about such definitions is that they are essentially functional in nature: they ask, can we operate in daily life, and without undue distress? In many ways, mental health is defined by the ability to fulfil a range of tasks and experience a range of emotions that we associate with 'normal' daily living (see *Table 1*, opposite).

The point of such definitions is that they emphasise the breadth of functioning across the normal events of life that can lead to sadness, anger or unhappiness, and that these are mentally healthy feelings as long as we can manage them and they do not become causes of social isolation or very prolonged distress. In this view of mental health, happiness is a state of mind that can occur but is by no means necessary to good mental health.

Table 1: Good mental health is…

The ability to….	
▓ Start, keep and, if necessary, end relationships	▓ Deal with what others think about you
▓ Work or attend college/school	▓ Accept failure and deal with success
▓ Look after oneself and others	▓ Function sexually, if wished
▓ Sleep	▓ Learn
▓ Laugh and cry	▓ Deal with loss
▓ Eat	▓ Express good feelings
▓ Avoid problems with substances	▓ Manage negative feelings

Models of mental illness

As implied above, many models of mental illness have existed over the centuries and a significant number continue to be current, and to affect policy and practice today (Colombo *et al*, 2003). These can be summarised as follows (Jenkins *et al*, 2002):

▓ biological models that are concerned with the biological and chemical basis of mental illness – this is fundamentally what we refer to as the 'medical model', although many doctors use a more integrative model (McCulloch *et al*, 2005)

▓ social/psychological models that are concerned with life events, family dynamics and belief systems or thinking style. This also encapsulates social models of disability that focus on how society reacts to the disabled individual, often in a discriminatory way, as well as the disability itself

▓ intuitive/spiritual explanations that see the mind as a battleground for conflicting forces: the unconscious v the conscious, good v evil etc. Psychoanalysis encapsulates this within modern western thinking, but belief in demonic possession is still prevalent in many societies

▓ existential belief, which views mental illness as another valid form of human existence – this is rarer.

Of course, some current models or belief systems are hybrids of more than one model: the recovery movement could be viewed as embracing both the social/psychological and the intuitive/spiritual, for example. These models are very important because they imply certain treatment mechanisms and social responses and determine how we respond to mental illness (see *Table 2*).

Table 2: Models of mental illness and treatment response

Model	Treatment/response
Biological	Medication, ECT
Social/psychological	Psychological interventions, social interventions
Intuitive	Psychoanalysis, exorcism
Existential	Acceptance

Why do so many models exist? It could be argued that the diversity of thinking about mental illness reflects the challenges it poses to our thinking and to our ability to respond as communities and societies. No one model has an absolute advantage in terms of the evidence base. The fact that psychiatric diagnosis is not highly reliable, and that many psychiatric symptoms are widely distributed in the general population (Bentall, 2003) leads us to question the biomedical model, as does the lack of disease-specific treatments. To put it another way, what is the value of a medical diagnosis if it cannot predict the outcome of the treatment? One could argue that a combination of the biological, psychological and social models fits the evidence base best, but it must be recognised that the models are all partly culturally determined (Spector, 2003). It is also interesting that outcomes for mental illness in developing countries are sometimes better than they are in the west, despite lack of medical and psychological interventions (Jablensky *et al*, 1992).

An overview of mental illness

A consideration of the different kinds of mental illness helps to illustrate some important points. The five major groups of mental illness are outlined in *Table 3* opposite.

These five groups represent significantly different phenomena with different associated genetic, family and social associations. While diagnosis is unreliable for many specific mental illnesses, it is clear that mental illness, however we label it, is a recognisable phenomenon across all nations and cultures and comes in recognisable patterns. However, sometimes these patterns overlap or change over time.

Common mental disorders, such as depression and anxiety disorders, are among the most important and troublesome conditions to affect mankind. Many have clear social and psychological precursors, such as adverse life events, but there may be genetic and family predispositions as well.

Table 3: The five major groups of mental illness

Group	Example
Common mental disorders (includes enduring common mental disorders)	Depression
Severe mental disorders	Schizophrenia
Substance misuse disorders	Alcohol related disorders
Abnormal personality traits ('personality disorders')	Antisocial personality disorder
Dementias	Alzheimer's disease

The severe mental disorders consist of bipolar (manic-depressive) illness, schizophrenia and anorexia. These may have a heavier genetic and family element as precursors. But it is important to know that some severe mental disorder is not enduring over time (20% of people with a diagnosis of schizophrenia only experience one breakdown), while some common disorders are enduring and disabling. In other words, diagnosis does not predict level of disability. All mental disorders can correlate with poorer physical health: for example, depression and schizophrenia are both linked with heart disease and type II diabetes.

Substance misuse disorders are, self-evidently, triggered by use of substances. This may involve excessive use (as in much alcoholism) or psychological vulnerability triggered by use (as in psychosis induced by cannabis), and usually both. They sometimes co-exist with severe or common mental disorders. Many people, particularly women, suffering from so-called dual diagnosis have been abused as children, as is the case in a number of other mental disorders.

Personality problems represent highly debatable territory and many practitioners reject the medical model for these disorders. Two thirds of the prison population would fit a diagnosis of personality disorder, which begs the question: what is the difference between criminality or deviance and personality disorder? Personality disorder is generally applied to people with dysfunctional patterns of behaviour that are established in early childhood and only seem to respond to long-term, intensive psychological treatments. People with this label are often rejected by mental health services as 'untreatable', although they can be very distressed or anxious and may benefit from emotional and behavioural interventions.

Finally, dementias are a progressive, degenerative brain disease. The causes are not fully known but can be genetic, environmental, and/or related to cardiac/circulatory problems and sometimes to brain injury and substance misuse. While the dementias differ from other disorders in that they are evidently diseases of the brain, they do have some features in common with other mental disorders, including risk factors and the association with physical health and cardiovascular disease in particular.

It can be seen that mental illnesses are varied and heterogeneous and that some of the models outlined above fit some illnesses better than others, which is another reason why the models are so varied. From a mental health perspective, the commonalities between mental illnesses are probably the most interesting. These include:

- feelings of guilt, shame, anxiety, fear and confusion commonly occur in most mental illnesses, at onset and as a result of the illness itself

- concurrent physical ill health is common

- risk factors such as lifetime anxiety, poor parenting, genetic predisposition, substance misuse and many others are shared across a range of illnesses, but we have to be careful about what 'causes' what

- most illnesses respond best to holistic treatments that combine medical, psychological, social and personal responses. Yet such integrated care is hardly ever available in statutory services.

The integrative approach

At one level, the biomedical model is faced with the same challenge as any other model used to explain mental health and illness. It is not the medical model or those who use it who must find a way forward; we all need to develop a fuller understanding of the different aspects of mental health and mental illness and how they relate to each other.

Although different models tap into different aspects of the human condition, practitioners need to view them as complementary rather than conflicting. For example, the medical model is concerned with an external, objective reality – looking from outside at the individual; the psychotherapeutic model is more interested in internal, subjective realities and our thoughts and feelings.

The various models can also be understood when they are grouped along two simple dimensions (subjective/objective and self/others) as shown in *Table 4* opposite.

Table 4: Dimensions of mental illness (after Wilber, 2000)

	Subjective	**Objective**
Individual/self	'I' Interior (Intervention eg. psychoanalysis)	'It' Exterior (Intervention eg. CBT, drugs)
Collective/self and others	'We' Interior collective (Intervention eg. group therapy)	'They' Exterior collective (Intervention eg. anti- bullying strategies in schools)

A strict biological interpretation of the medical model positions it in the upper right quadrant of the figure, which is only a part of human experience. This suggests there are clear limits to the usefulness of the medical model in understanding mental illness and especially mental health. If we want to conceptualise all aspects of mental health, whether as public policy makers, practitioners or just citizens, we need to think about all four quadrants of the figure.

An integrated future also depends on non-medical practitioners being aware of the limits of their own influence. The objective is not to eradicate the medical model but to make it part of an integrated understanding of mental health and illness. This is not to say we should stop specialising in psychiatry, psychology, medicine or other disciplines. Instead, we should acknowledge that our specialist knowledge is vital, but partial. From this position we will be better placed to provide holistic, integrated care by joining with others: those who have complementary specialist knowledge, and those who have reflected on their own lived experience or delivered practical help to others. An integrated approach will also provide people with mental health problems with more choice, both when developing their own understanding of their mental health and when choosing the most appropriate and preferred interventions, including self-management and self-help initiatives.

Acknowledgment
With thanks to Iain Ryrie, director of mental health research at the Mental Health Foundation, for his helpful comments.

References

Bentall RP (2003) *Madness explained: psychosis and human nature.* London: Allen Lane/Penguin Press.

Colombo A, Bendelow G, Fulford KWM *et al* (2003) Evaluating the influence of implicit models of mental disorder on processes of shared decision-making within community-based multidisciplinary teams. *Social Science & Medicine* **56** 1557-1570.

Jablensky A, Sartorius N, Ensberg G *et al* (1992) Schizophrenia: manifestations, incidence and cause in different cultures – a World Health Organisation ten country study. *Psychological Medicine Monograph* **s20** 1-97.

Jenkins R, McCulloch A, Friedli L *et al* (2002) *Developing a national mental health policy.* Maudsley monograph 43. Hove: The Psychology Press.

Layard R (2005) *Happiness: lessons from a new science.* Harmondsworth: Penguin Press.

McCulloch A, Ryrie I, Williamson T *et al* (2005) The medical model: has it a future? *Mental Health Review* **10** (1) 7-15.

Spector RE (2003) *Cultural diversity in health and illness.* New Jersey: Prentice Hall.

Wilber K (2000) *Sex, ecology and spirituality: the spirit of evolution.* Boston: Shambhala.

World Health Organisation (1946) *Constitution.* Geneva: WHO.

Chapter 2
Public mental health and mental health promotion

Lynne Friedli

'Transforming the NHS from a sickness service to a health service is not just a matter of promoting physical health. Understanding how everyone in the NHS can promote mental well-being is equally important.' (Department of Health, 2004)

In 1999 the government published its national service framework (NSF) for mental health, setting explicit targets for work to improve mental health and prevent mental illness (Department of Health, 1999). Standard 1 of the NSF explicitly requires mental health and social services to:

- 'promote mental health for all, working with individuals and communities
- 'combat discrimination against individuals and groups with mental health problems, and promote their social inclusion.'

Traditionally, mental health promotion has been a low priority for both the mental health and public health sectors. Progress towards achieving even the basic building blocks for standard 1 has been notably slow (Appleby, 2004). But this is changing, partly due to a much greater emphasis at national policy level on the promotion and prevention role of the NHS (Department of Health, 2004; Wanless, 2002; 2004), and also in response to a growing body of evidence that positive mental health is inextricably linked with improved physical health and health choices, better quality of life and personal relationships, reduced crime, higher educational attainment, and employability. These are all key themes in the public health white paper Choosing Health (Department of Health, 2004), in Our Health, Our Care, Our Say (Department of Health, 2006), and in Making it Possible (NIMHE, 2005), which provides a framework for the delivery of standard 1 of the NSF.

More broadly, mental health promotion also intersects with current debates about happiness, well-being and quality of life, and their relevance to social and economic policy making (Huppert *et al*, 2005; Layard, 2005; Marks & Shah, 2004; Seligman, 2003). This chapter outlines the relevance and importance of mental health promotion for practitioners working in a wide range of settings across all sectors, and covers the following themes:

- defining mental health and mental health promotion
- determinants of mental health
- impact of mental health on wider health and social outcomes
- mental health promotion interventions
- mental health indicators.

What's in a name?

Mental health promotion is essentially concerned with:

- how individuals, families, organisations and communities think and feel
- the factors that influence how we think and feel, individually and collectively
- the impact that this has on overall health and well-being. (Friedli, 2000).

Although, in practice, mental health promotion interventions often focus on prevention, there is general agreement that mental health is more than the absence of mental illness:

> 'Everyone has mental health needs, whether or not they have a diagnosis. These needs are met, or not met, at home, in families, at work, on the streets, in schools and neighbourhoods, in prisons and hospitals – where people feel respected, included and safe, or on the margins, in fear and excluded.' (Department of Health, 2001)

> 'Mental health is the emotional and spiritual resilience which allows us to enjoy life and to survive pain, disappointment and sadness. It is a positive sense of well-being and an underlying belief in our own and others' dignity and worth.' (Health Education Authority, 1997)

The definition of mental health as a 'positive sense of well-being' challenges the idea that mental health is the opposite of mental illness and is generally referred to as the 'two factors model', with mental health and mental illness conceptualised as separate continua (Keyes, 2005). While there is a tendency for mental health to improve as mental illness symptoms decrease, research suggests this relationship is modest. Someone with a diagnosis of schizophrenia might nevertheless feel supported, at ease and optimistic. They might be coping well with life and enjoying a high level of well-being. This is a significant aspect of the recovery agenda, which shifts the focus from mental illness services to the wider community and asks what a person needs to regain or hold on to a life that has meaning for them (Bates, 2002; Sayce, 2002; Perkins, 2002). Equally, many people who do not have a clinical diagnosis have low levels of mental health (Gilleard *et al*, 2005) and might benefit from an environment that actively promotes positive mental well-being.

The case for mental health promotion is based on the known relationship between good mental health (which is a worthwhile end in itself), and improved outcomes for:

- physical health
- education
- employment
- parenting
- relationships
- crime
- health behaviours
- quality of life.

Mental well-being protects physical health and improves health outcomes and recovery rates, notably for coronary heart disease, stroke and diabetes. Poor mental health significantly increases the risk of poor physical health and is associated with poor self-management of chronic illness and a range of health-damaging behaviours, including smoking, drug and alcohol abuse, unwanted pregnancy and poor diet. Stress epidemiology demonstrates the link between feelings of despair, anger, frustration, hopelessness, low self-worth and higher cholesterol levels, blood pressure and susceptibility to infection (Marmot & Wilkinson, 2006). For heart disease, psychosocial factors are on a par with the more widely recognised risk factors of smoking, high blood pressure, obesity and cholesterol problems.

Many people have symptoms of mental distress that do not reach clinical levels but, for both clinical and non-clinical populations, even small improvements in mental well-being contribute to improved physical health, productivity and quality of life. Self-reported health status correlates more closely with life satisfaction than objective health status, suggesting that mental health is an important mediator of overall health.

While there may be broad agreement that improving mental well-being is a worthwhile goal, there is far less consensus on the ethics and potential consequences of a prevention agenda. If the goal of interventions is to eliminate all disorders of the mind, this raises human rights and civil liberties issues. In the same way that the disability rights movement challenges the goal of seeking to eradicate all conditions that result in physical disabilities, questions need to be asked about issues of conformity and diversity that have important implications for mental health policy and practice.

Determinants of mental health

Mental health promotion is one element of a population-wide approach to understanding and addressing risk and protective factors for mental health and well-being, described as public mental health:

> 'Public mental health… provides a strategic and analytical framework for addressing the wider determinants of mental health, reducing the enduring inequalities in the distribution of mental distress and improving the mental health of the whole population.' (Friedli, 2004)

'Public mental health might be called the science, art and politics of creating a mentally healthy society.' (Friedli, 2004)

The focus on mental health as a public health issue is linked to the renaissance of interest in public health following publication of the Wanless reports, which were commissioned by the Treasury to provide evidence of the economic advantages of investment in prevention of ill health (Wanless, 2002; 2004). However, it is also evidence of a growing recognition that mental health influences physical health, health outcomes for a wide range of diseases (including coronary heart disease, type II diabetes and cancer) and the extent to which people feel able and motivated to exercise choice and control and to adopt healthy lifestyles.

'How people feel is not an elusive or abstract concept, but a significant public health indicator; as significant as rates of smoking, obesity and physical activity.' (Department of Health, 2001)

One of the most significant debates about public mental health concerns the balance between interventions that focus on strengthening individuals, and those that address the wider determinants of mental health. It has been argued that focusing on 'emotional resilience' or 'life skills', for example, may imply that people should learn to cope with deprivation and disadvantage (Secker, 1998).

Recognition of the socio-economic and environmental determinants of mental well-being has led to a growing emphasis on models that work at different levels – for example:

- strengthening individuals – by increasing emotional resilience through interventions designed to promote self-esteem, life and coping skills, eg. communicating, negotiating, relationship and parenting skills

- strengthening communities – by increasing social support, social inclusion and participation, improving community safety, neighbourhood environments, promoting childcare and self-help networks, developing health and social services that support mental health, improving mental health within schools and workplaces, eg. through anti-bullying strategies and mental health strategies

- reducing structural barriers to mental health – through initiatives to reduce discrimination and inequalities and to promote access to education, meaningful employment, housing, services and support for those who are vulnerable. (Health Education Authority, 1997; Department of Health, 2001)

'Reducing structural barriers to mental health and introducing policies which protect mental well-being will benefit those who do and those who do not currently have mental health problems, and the many people who move between periods of mental health and mental illness.' (Department of Health, 2001)

Mental illness is not a random misfortune, but the product of social, economic, environmental and lifestyle factors that are well understood (Rogers & Pilgrim, 2003). Mental health status is strongly associated with material deprivation: education, employment and the environment are key factors that influence which one in four of us is most at risk of mental health problems, across the spectrum of disorders. As with physical health, the poorest and most deprived families bear the main burden of mental distress. Lone parents, people with physical illnesses and the unemployed make up 20% of the population, but these three groups constitute 36% of all those with neurotic disorders, 39% of those with a limiting mental disorder and 51% of those with disabling mental disorders (Melzer *et al*, 2004). Other adverse life events that increase risk include being a carer, workplace stress, bereavement and bullying. There is also increasingly robust evidence for an association between lifestyle behaviours and mental health status and outcomes. These include physical activity, diet, alcohol consumption and the use of cannabis and other psychotropic substances (Mental Health Foundation 2006; 2005a; 2005b).

Interventions

Interventions to promote mental health and well-being include a very wide range of activities in a wide range of settings. They might include, for example, home visits to new mothers by health visitors or 'community mothers' to support parenting skills; anti bullying policies in schools, and adoption in workplaces of the HSE stress management guidelines and provision of counselling and talking therapies for employees experiencing stress at work or personal difficulties. For people with a diagnosed mental illness, interventions might include supported employment schemes, socially inclusive projects using mainstream sports and leisure facilities, provision of meaningful activities on acute wards, and befriending and suicide prevention schemes in the community. For older people, some areas have introduced befriending schemes and regular home visits, as well as group activities and arts and education projects to address isolation and give a purpose to their day. At a neighbourhood and community level, they could include crime and safety initiatives, noise abatement measures and provision of green open spaces. At a national level, activities may include campaigns to improve media coverage of mental illness, national government guidelines and standards for schools and workplaces and, more controversially, taxation and other fiscal policies aimed at reducing inequalities in income and child poverty, government interventions to boost local economies, or legislation that sets clear limits on density of housing.

There is currently no system for mapping mental health promotion activity, although (under standard 1 of the national service framework) all primary care trusts must have a local mental health promotion strategy (see NIMHE, 2005).

To date, tackling the discrimination and social exclusion experienced by people with a mental health diagnosis has tended to receive a stronger focus than promoting mental health for all (Social Exclusion Unit, 2004; NIMHE, 2005; Department of Health,

2004). Although the reform of mental illness services and addressing the deprivation of human rights and civil liberties experienced by people with mental health problems remain important goals, they are now also being considered in the context of public mental health. This is an important development because the focus on stigma and discrimination has tended to preclude a wider debate about factors that are toxic to mental health, whether or not one has a diagnosis. We have a wealth of data on public attitudes to mental illness (Gale *et al*, 2004; Braunholtz *et al*, 2004), but very little on public knowledge of what harms and hinders mental well-being.

Publication of Making it Possible (NIMHE, 2005) can be seen as an effort to achieve this broader focus and to provide greater leadership and support for a population-wide approach to improving mental health. Making it Possible identifies nine priorities for action to improve mental health (see *Table 1* opposite).

Measuring success

A major challenge for mental health promotion is defining the key elements or indicators of mental health and creating scales that can measure the mental health (as opposed to the mental illness) of individuals and populations (Parkinson, 2006). A shift in focus from measuring prevalence of psychiatric morbidity to capturing levels of mental health and well-being in populations has the potential to radically transform the way we think about mental health. It also creates new opportunities to consider the mental health impact of social and economic policy and to add a new dimension to political debate about future economic and social policy, at a national and global level.

Keyes and others have argued that positive mental health is a combination of positive feelings (subjective well-being) and positive functioning (engagement and fulfilment) (Keyes, 2002; Huppert, 2005). Measures are needed that can capture the range of emotional and cognitive attributes associated with a self-reported sense of well-being (Hird, 2003; McAllister, 2005). At an individual level they might include self-esteem, internal locus of control or mastery, resilience, satisfaction with life, optimism, social integration, sense of coherence and satisfying relationships (Huppert, 2005). At a community level they might include access to social support and safety; at a structural level, they might include equity of income and opportunity and access to public services.

Conclusion

The central tenet of mental health promotion is that everyone has mental health needs, whether or not they have a mental illness diagnosis, just as everyone has physical health needs, whether or not they are ill. It is widely recognised that physical well-being is a resource to be promoted through a combination of legislation, policy, education and fiscal measures. Mental health promotion aims to achieve the same recognition for mental health.

Table 1: Promoting mental health: key areas and measures of success

ACTION	MEASURES OF SUCCESS
Marketing mental health	▪ People are well informed and motivated to look after their own and others' mental health ▪ People have positive and accepting attitudes to people with mental health problems
Equality and inclusion	▪ People have access to a wide range of sources of support for emotional and psychological difficulties ▪ Reduction in inequalities in access to non-pharmacological sources of support, notably for black and minority ethnic communities and older people
Tackling violence and abuse	▪ Reduction in prevalence of mental health problems ▪ Reduction in self-harming behaviour
Parents and early years	▪ Parents and care-givers have the knowledge, skills and capacity to meet the emotional and social needs of infants and young children ▪ Parents and carers have access to support for themselves and their parenting roles, delivered in a way that is evidence based and meets their needs
Schools	▪ Schools achieving National Healthy Schools targets[1] and delivering SEAL[2]
Employment	▪ Reduction in mental health-related unemployment
Workplace	▪ Workplaces adopt HSE stress management standards ▪ Support to enable people off work with mental health problems to return to work
Communities	▪ Improved quality of life and life satisfaction ▪ Increase in the proportion of local areas with a high 'liveability' score
Later life	▪ Improved life satisfaction among older people ▪ Increased opportunities for older people to participate

(NIMHE, 2005)

[1] See www.wiredforhealth.gov.uk

[2] Social and Emotional Aspects of Learning. See http://publications.teachernet.gov.uk

References

Appleby L (2004) *National service framework for mental health – five years on.* London: Department of Health.

Bates P (ed) (2002) *Working for inclusion: making social inclusion a reality for people with severe mental health problems.* London: Sainsbury Centre for Mental Health.

Braunholtz S, Davidson S, King S (2004) *Well? What do you think (2004)? The second national Scottish survey of public attitudes to mental health, mental well-being and mental health problems.* Edinburgh: Scottish Executive Social Research. (www.scotland.gov.uk/Publications/2005/01/20506/49641)

Department of Health (1999) *National service framework for mental health: modern standards and service models.* London: Department of Health.

Department of Health (2001) *Making it happen: a guide to delivering mental health promotion.* London: Department of Health. (www.doh.gov.uk/index.htm)

Department of Health (2004) *Choosing health: making healthy choices easier.* London: Department of Health.

Department of Health (2006) *Our health, our care, our say: a new direction for community services.* London: Department of Health. www.dh.gov.uk/assetRoot/04/12/74/59/04127459.pdf

Friedli L (2000) Mental health promotion: rethinking the evidence base. *Mental Health Review* **5** (3) 15-18.

Friedli L (2004) Editorial. *Journal of Mental Health Promotion* **3** (1) 2-6.

Gale E, Seymour L, Crepaz-Keay D *et al* (2004) *Scoping review on mental health anti-stigma and discrimination – current activities and what works.* Leeds: NIMHE.

Gilleard C, Pond C, Scammell A *et al* (2005) Well-being in Wandsworth: a public mental health audit. *Journal of Public Mental Health* **4** (2) 14-22.

Health Education Authority (1997) *Mental health promotion: a quality framework.* London: HEA.

Hird S (2003) *What is wellbeing? A brief review of current literature and concepts.* Edinburgh: NHS Scotland. (www.phis.org.uk/doc.pl?file=pdf/What%20is%20wellbeing%202.doc)

Huppert FA, Baylis N, Keverne B (eds) (2005) *The science of well-being.* Oxford: Oxford University Press.

Keyes CLM (2002) The mental health continuum: from languishing to flourishing in life. *Journal of Health and Social Research* **43** 207-222.

Keyes CLM (2005) Mental illness and/or mental health? Investigating axioms of the complete state model of health. *Journal of Consulting and Clinical Psychology* **73** 539-548.

Layard R (2005) *Happiness: lessons from a new science.* London: Allen Lane.

Marks N, Shah H (2004) A well-being manifesto for a flourishing society. *Journal of Mental Health Promotion* **3** (4) 9-15.

Marmot M, Wilkinson RG (2006) *Social determinants of health.* Oxford: Oxford University Press.

McAllister F (2005) *Wellbeing concepts and challenges: discussion paper.* London: Sustainable Development Research Network. (www.sd-research.org.uk/documents/ SDRNwellbeingpaperfinal-20December2005_v3_000.pdf)

Melzer D, Fryers T, Jenkins R (eds) (2004) *Social inequalities and the distribution of common mental disorders.* Maudsley monograph 44. Hove: Psychology Press.

Mental Health Foundation (2005a) *Up and running? Exercise therapy and the treatment of mild or moderate depression in primary care.* London: Mental Health Foundation.

Mental Health Foundation (2005b) *Choosing mental health: a policy agenda for mental health and public health.* London: Mental Health Foundation.

Mental Health Foundation (2006) *Feeding minds: the impact of food on mental health.* London: Mental Health Foundation.

NIMHE (2005) *Making it possible: improving mental health and well-being in England.* Leeds: NIMHE/CSIP. (http://kc.nimhe.org.uk/upload/making%20it%20possible%20Final%20pdf1.pdf)

Parkinson J (2006) Establishing a core set of sustainable national mental health and well-being indicators for Scotland. *Journal of Public Mental Health* **5** (1) 42-48.

Perkins R (2002) Are you (really) being served? *Mental Health Today* (September) 18-21.

Rogers A, Pilgrim D (2003) *Mental health and inequality.* Basingstoke: Palgrave.

Sayce L (2002) Inclusion as a new paradigm: civil rights. In: Bates P (ed) *Working for inclusion: making social inclusion a reality for people with severe mental health problems.* London: Sainsbury Centre for Mental Health.

Secker J(1998) Current conceptualisations of mental health and mental health promotion. *Health Education Research* **13** (1) 57-66.

Seligman M (2003) *Authentic happiness: using the new positive psychology to realize your potential for lasting fulfilment.* Cambridge: Simon and Schuster.

Social Exclusion Unit (2004) *Mental health and social exclusion.* London: Office of the Deputy Prime Minister.

Wanless D (2002) *Securing our future health: taking a long-term view.* London: Stationery Office.

Wanless D (2004) *Securing good health for the whole population: final report.* London: HM Treasury. (www.hm treasury.gov.uk/wanless)

Chapter 3
Building bridges to social inclusion

Louise Lingwood

In broad terms, social inclusion refers to the degree to which individuals, families and community groups are able to participate in society. Poverty, discrimination and disadvantage can exclude individuals, groups and whole communities from realising their potential. Barriers to inclusion include family breakdown, low skills, unemployment, low income, poor housing and ill health. Social groups that have been identified by the government as particularly vulnerable to exclusion include the unemployed, lone parents, disabled people, people facing discrimination on the grounds of gender, race or sexuality, homeless people, people with few qualifications, people with low self-esteem, people with addiction problems and whole communities in areas of deprivation (SEU, 2004a).

People with mental health problems

People with disabilities have historically been located towards the edges of community life, rather than in the main flow. People who experience mental health problems are among the most excluded of all social groups. It has been estimated that, at best, some 20% of people of working age with severe mental health problems are employed: significantly fewer than in other disabled groups (SEU, 2004b). The Social Exclusion Unit, in its report on mental health (SEU, 2004b), identified a number of reasons why. First and foremost there is widespread stigma and discrimination against people with mental health problems. Indeed, it is argued that they are the most stigmatised of all people with disabilities (Thornicroft, 2006). The SEU report found that, despite campaigns aimed at tackling stigma, more than six out of ten employers would not recruit someone with a mental health problem. Negative media coverage of mental health issues is regarded by many mental health service users as influencing public perceptions. In a survey by the mental health charity Mind, 73% of the 515 respondents complained that media coverage was increasingly negative and biased; half said that media coverage had a negative effect on their mental health; 24% said they had experienced hostility from their neighbours and local communities as a result of media reports, and 22% said their family and friends had reacted negatively to them because of recent media coverage of mental health issues (Mind, 2000). It is not surprising, then, that people with mental health problems frequently have concerns about disclosing their condition, even to friends and family.

People from black and minority ethnic (BME) communities who have mental health problems are particularly at risk. They are six times more likely than white people to be detained under the Mental Health Act (Healthcare Commission, 2005), and are more likely to seek professional help at a much later stage, when problems can be more severe. They are also more likely to experience multiple deprivations and inequalities of income, employment, physical health and other socio-economic factors known to have a negative impact on mental health and to be associated with social exclusion (SEU, 2004c).

Social networks and housing

Sayce (2001) describes a complex relationship between social exclusion and mental ill health. Many of the factors that can cause exclusion, like low income, lack of social networks, poor health and unemployment, can be both the cause of and an outcome of mental ill health, and people can find themselves caught in a cycle of exclusion. A lack of strong social networks, for example, can have a negative impact on mental well-being, and their presence can positively influence the recovery process. Mental illness can be a very lonely experience. A Mind (2004) survey found that 84% of people with mental health problems report feeling isolated, compared with 29% of the general population. Young people, people from ethnic minorities and people in rural communities were found to be most vulnerable to isolation. A common consequence of mental ill health can be the loss of contact with family and friends: for example, divorce and separation rates among people with psychotic disorders stand at 47%, compared with 22% in the general population (Singleton *et al*, 2001). As a result, many people find that their social networks are limited to other people in the mental health system.

Alongside positive social networks, access to stable housing is fundamental to mental well-being and a general sense of security, and is essential if people are to participate in work and community life. Four out of five people considered to have a severe and enduring mental health problem live in mainstream housing. They are much more likely to live in rented accommodation than the general population, and are twice as likely to say they are dissatisfied with their living arrangements. One in four will have serious rent arrears and face eviction (SEU, 2004b). Not surprisingly, such factors can have a serious negative impact on a person's mental health. People with mental health problems who are homeless can be considered as having a 'priority need' under current legislation, although many will be placed in temporary bed and breakfast before securing more settled accommodation.

Promoting social inclusion

People thrive best when the fullness of community participation is open to them. This is explicitly recognised in current government policy on mental health day care and vocational support. The growing trend towards 'day services without walls' (London Development Centre, 2005) is shaping a wealth of new social, educational and vocational services that aim to 'mainstream' activities, supported by Department of Health commissioning guidance (NIMHE/CSIP, 2006a; 2006b).

The starting point for mental health workers wishing to maximise social inclusion is to embrace practices that facilitate recovery and inclusion. Adopting the recovery approach is key to increasing social inclusion opportunities. It is an approach that is profoundly influenced by people's expectations and attitudes, and calls for a substantial degree of optimism and commitment from all concerned. Recovery does not necessarily mean getting back to where the individual was before. The approach recognises that recovery happens in fits and starts and, like life, has many ups and downs (Wallcraft, 2005). Adopted as a key value in the 2006 review of mental health nursing (Department of Health, 2006), the recovery approach requires person-centred plans that reflect the individual's aspirations and priorities, and looks beyond mental health services to explore opportunities in the wider community. Person-centred planning focuses on how an individual wants to live their life and what is required to make that possible, building on individual strengths and experience.

Access to mainstream opportunities

One of the primary aims of mental health workers should be to provide a supportive bridge between the individual and mainstream opportunities in the wider community. This involves them in mapping and engaging with local community resources outside specialist mental health services, such as leisure facilities and opportunities for volunteering, education and training. There is evidence of a positive connection between physical exercise and mental well-being (Mental Health Foundation, 2005), and there now exists a number of schemes whereby GPs can write a prescription for people to attend leisure centres and gyms. Many local authorities now run 'green gyms', bringing people together to enjoy local walks or take part in conservation projects, for example. People with mental health problems frequently cite the cost of accessing leisure facilities as their main reason for not using them. Mental health workers can help their clients negotiate discounts, access direct payments to pay for entry fees, and obtain exercise on prescription. This role may be particularly appropriate for day service workers, who can act as a bridge to a wide range of mainstream community opportunities (see, for example, Carr, 2005).

Fewer than one in three people with mental health problems have any formal qualifications. The low confidence of service users, complicated enrolment procedures, inflexible courses that do not take account of fluctuating health conditions, and lack of money to cover fees, transport and books etc are just some of the difficulties people experience when attempting to access mainstream education (SEU, 2004b). However, further education institutions are obliged under the Disability Discrimination Act to ensure access to all sections of the community, and mental health workers can ease access to mainstream courses by engaging the support of college tutors and fellow students. Partnerships developed between mental health service providers and colleges, for example, have created stepping-stones to mainstream education and training. Typically this takes three forms: discrete programmes, especially designed for people with mental health problems; integrated programmes, where people with mental health problems participate in mainstream classes, and a combination of the two, where people with mental health problems take a discrete programme as a precursor to, or in parallel with, a mainstream course.

Volunteering is another route to engagement with the mainstream. Volunteering can help counter isolation and offer individuals the chance to make a contribution to society. In London, for example, the Capital Volunteering Scheme brings together the statutory and voluntary sectors to offer a wide range of part-time and full-time volunteering opportunities, many user led, including 'time banks', where participants offer their own skills in return for the skills and services of others. Volunteering can increase self-worth, develop vocational and interpersonal skills and boost confidence. For those wanting to return to work, it can be a useful route to employment (Ellis & Davis Smith, 2004).

Employment and job retention

Work plays a central role in our lives. The majority of people with mental health problems would like paid employment, or at least to engage in some kind of meaningful work. Being employed has an important role both in maintaining mental health and promoting recovery, and is a key factor in social inclusion. Indeed, the high rates of unemployment among people with mental illness are thought to be associated more with social factors than with the disabilities of the illness itself (House of Commons Work and Pensions Committee, 2003).

For people in work when they become ill, early access to employment advice and support is extremely important in helping them maintain and return to their job, which in turn can have a positive impact on their confidence and recovery (Rinaldi *et al*, 2006). CMHTs, day services and other rehabilitative services have a central role in helping people maintain or access employment (NIMHE/CSIP, 2006a). Standard 5 of the national service framework for mental health (Department of Health, 1999) requires that the care plans of all people on enhanced CPA should demonstrate how suitable employment or other occupational activity will be secured. However low expectations among some mental health workers are perceived as an obstacle to individual aspiration. Furthermore, CMHTs typically have few links with employment agencies and employers, and few include workers with the specialist vocational knowledge and skills needed to assist people getting into work. The Department of Health guidance on commissioning vocational opportunities for people with severe mental illness (NIMHE/CSIP, 2006a) recognises this problem and recommends the employment of vocational specialists in clinical teams. One approach that is recognised to be particularly effective is IPS (individual placement support), which places people in work and provides ongoing support, rather than training them for jobs that may not be available. Support is also provided to the employer to help maintain the placement.

While the evidence clearly backs the development of supported employment placements, there are other models of employment services. Some see the development of social firms as the possible solution to providing sheltered work. Social firms aspire to be successful businesses and may offer a positive replacement for outdated 'sheltered employment' schemes.

Social inclusion skills

While current mental health training may include aspects of social inclusion, there is a perception at national level of the need to ensure the training of mental health workers focuses on social outcomes and equips them with the necessary competencies to promote individual recovery and social inclusion. The ten 'essential shared capabilities' (Department of Health, 2004a) are widely recognised as the core skills that all mental health professionals should possess, and many of these capabilities focus on recovery and inclusion.

The ten essential shared capabilities:

1   Working in partnership
2   Respecting diversity
3   Practising ethically
4   Challenging inequality
5   Promoting recovery
6   Identifying people's needs and strengths
7   Providing service user-centred care
8   Making a difference
9   Promoting safety and positive risk taking
10 Personal development and learning

Progress towards achieving a mental health workforce able to deliver the kinds of mental services and interventions required in the 21st century has seen the emergence of new roles such as support, time, recovery (STR) workers, carer support workers, graduate and gateway primary mental health care workers and community development workers, for example, that embrace many of these competencies (Appleby, 2004). In the voluntary sector, community bridge builders and employment support and retention workers are new roles that are having a significant impact on delivering the social inclusion agenda (London Development Centre, 2005).

Service development and social inclusion

Alongside the development of new competencies and workforce roles to deliver social inclusion, it is crucial that the way in which we provide services is also reviewed. It is essential that service development involves service users, and explores the potential for user-led services. For example, mental health services should involve people from BME communities in the design and delivery of services. Of necessity this will require the involvement of people from those communities in the design process and the engagement of community and faith groups in the delivery of services. There is both a responsibility and a need for sectors outside the specialist mental health services to promote social inclusion and it is anticipated that cross-sector working will play an important part in delivering services that support recovery and provide mainstream opportunities. There is already evidence of new partnership working delivering innovative, community-based day services, for example.

The voluntary sector is currently perceived as having the flexibility to respond more quickly to changes in demand for service delivery, and to the specialist needs of particular minority groups (most notably, people from BME communities) (Department of Health, 2005). Indeed, the Department of Health expressly requires that the voluntary sector be viewed by NHS commissioners as equal partners in the delivery of mental health services (Department of Health, 2004b), and most recently has taken the further step of establishing a Social Enterprise Unit with the aim to support and encourage entrepreneurialism in the provision of health and social care.

Thus achieving social inclusion and positive social outcomes for people with mental health problems can be seen as the main drivers of current mental health service development. The aim is to break down the metaphorical walls that still divide people with mental health problems from the rest of society and their communities by preventing their drift towards the edges of society and into a 'psychiatric career', and initiating interventions to enable their re-engagement at as early a point as possible following their entry into treatment.

References

Appleby L (2004) *National service framework for mental health – five years on.* London: Department of Health.

Carr M (2005) Bridge-building with Mainstream. *A Life in the Day* **9** (4) 15-19.

Department of Health (1999) *National service framework for mental health: modern standards and service models.* London: Department of Health.

Department of Health (2004a) *The ten essential shared capabilities: a framework for the whole of the mental health workforce.* London: Department of Health.

Department of Health (2004b) *Making partnership work for patients, carers and service users: a strategic agreement between the Department of Health, the NHS and the voluntary and community sector.* London: Department of Health.

Department of Health (2005) *Delivering race equality in mental health care: an action plan for reform inside and outside services and the government's response to the independent inquiry into the death of David Bennett.* London: Department of Health.

Department of Health (2006) *From values to action: the Chief Nursing Officer's review of mental health nursing.* London: Department of Health.

Ellis A, Davis Smith J (2004) A sense of purpose. *Mental Health Today* (February) 20-23.

Healthcare Commission (2005). *Count me in: results of a national census of inpatients in mental health hospitals and facilities in England and Wales.* London: Healthcare Commission.

House of Commons Work and Pensions Committee (2003) *Employment for all: interim report.* London: the Stationery Office.

London Development Centre for Mental Health (2005) *Redesigning day services: a modernisation toolkit for London.* London: London Development Centre for Mental Health/Mental Health Foundation.

Mental Health Foundation (2005) *Up and running: exercise therapy and the treatment of mild or moderate depression in primary care.* London: Mental Health Foundation.

Mind (2000) *Counting the cost.* London: Mind.

Mind (2004) *Not alone? isolation and mental distress.* London: Mind.

NIMHE/CSIP (2006a) *Vocational services for people with severe mental health problems: commissioning guidance.* London: Department of Health.

NIMHE/CSIP (2006b) *From segregation to inclusion: commissioning guidance on day services for people with mental health problems.* London: Department of Health.

Rinaldi M, Perkins R, Hardisty J *et al* (2006) Not just stacking shelves. *A Life in the Day* **10** (1) 8-14.

Sayce L (2001) Social exclusion and mental health. *Psychiatric Bulletin* **25** 121-123.

SEU (2004a) *Breaking the cycle: taking stock of progress and priorities for the future.* London: Office of the Deputy Prime Minister.

SEU (2004b) *Mental health and social exclusion.* London: Office of the Deputy Prime Minister.

SEU (2004c) *Mental health and ethnicity.* Factsheet 8. London: Office of the Deputy Prime Minister.

Singleton N, Bumpstead R, O'Brien M *et al* (2001) *Psychiatric morbidity among adults living in private households, 2000.* London: the Stationery Office.

Thornicroft G (2006) *Actions speak louder: tackling discrimination against people with mental illness.* London: Mental Health Foundation.

Wallcraft J (2005) Recovery from mental breakdown. In: Tew J (ed) *Social perspectives in mental health.* London: Jessica Kingsley Publishers.

Chapter 4
Breaking the spiral of oppression: racism and race equality in the mental health system

Frank Keating

The needs, issues and concerns of black[1] and minority ethnic people (BME) with mental health problems have been pushed to the fore of the national health policy agenda (Department of Health, 1999; Department of Health, 2005). It has been acknowledged that achieving good mental health care for individuals from these communities is one of the biggest challenges for mental health services in England and Wales (Healthcare Commission, 2005) because of the disparities in rates of mental illness, treatment, care and outcomes. Explanations for this seemingly intractable situation are mixed and varied. This chapter will explore the complexities involved when we link mental illness with issues of 'race', culture and ethnicity and will make suggestions for addressing these in mental health practice. It will specifically focus on the issues of diversity and (in)equality pertaining to 'race' and ethnicity for visible minorities. This is not to deny the fact that there are also disparities for other minority ethnic groups, such as the Irish.

Mental illness and 'race' are contested areas of knowledge. A range of social, political and moral discourses come into play when these constructs are linked for analysis and understanding. For example, we encounter debates about definitions and causes of madness and the most effective treatments for it; discourses about identity – in particular, racialised identities; discourses about 'race' and its cluster of subcomponents (ethnicity, culture, etc), and discourses about domination, subordination, colonialism, slavery, resistance and inequality. This chapter will start with a brief overview of the current situation for BME communities in the UK and highlight some of the disparities in mental health.

Setting the context

Britain is a multi-ethnic and multi-cultural society where the percentage of the population that is from minority groups is steadily increasing. In 2001 minority groups comprised seven per cent of the population, with a concentration in London and other inner city areas. BME communities occupy particular positions of disadvantage in the

---

[1] The term 'black' will be used as a shorthand to refer to people of African, Asian and Caribbean origin, but this is not to deny the heterogeneity in and between these communities.

UK. Inequalities are reflected across all indices of economic and social well-being (White, 2002). They generally have higher rates of unemployment, live in poorer housing, report poorer health, have lower levels of academic achievement and higher rates of exclusions from schools and are over-represented in prison statistics.

This bleak picture is replicated when one considers the evidence for mental health. The 2005 census of inpatient services in England and Wales (Healthcare Commission, 2005) found in relation to BME communities:

- less involvement of general practitioners in referrals to mental health services
- greater involvement of police in referrals
- higher rates of referrals to mental health services by the courts
- greater likelihood of being detained under the Mental Health Act 1983
- higher rates of detention in medium and high secure wards
- higher rates of control and restraint.

Why this is so, the report concludes, is still not fully known. Some have sought biological explanations for these disparities; others have looked for social explanations (Morgan *et al*, 2004), while others offer racism as a causal factor (Fernando, 2003; McKenzie, 2002). However, none of these hypotheses have fully explained why black people have been so disproportionately exposed to the harsher, more restrictive end of the mental health system over the last 30 years. For example, to suggest that racism based on skin colour is a causal factor does not explain the mental health disparities for Irish communities in England (Pilgrim, 2005). Evidence shows that rates of schizophrenia for the Irish are second to those in African-Caribbean communities (Bracken *et al*, 1998). Life stressors have also been suggested as a causal factor, but Gilvarry *et al* (1999) found no differences in life stressors between white and BME groups, although they did find that black people tend to attribute adverse life events to racism.

A tragic but significant marker for BME communities was the death of David (Rocky) Bennett while being restrained by nursing staff on a medium secure ward. After a long campaign by his family, an independent inquiry report concluded that the NHS mental health services are 'institutionally racist' (Norfolk, Suffolk and Cambridgeshire SHA, 2003). The government subsequently published an action plan for Delivering Race Equality (DRE) (Department of Health, 2005). This plan has three building blocks:

- to develop more appropriate and responsive services

- to provide better quality information on the mental health needs of BME communities

- to encourage greater community engagement in the planning and delivery of mental health services.

Laudable as these intentions are, they contain a number of weaknesses. DRE focuses on organisational change, but fails to appreciate the heterogeneity within the BME population, and the complex range of identities and practices it contains (Bhui *et al*, 2004). It also fails to appreciate that the inequalities in mental health for black people exist within a broader historical and contemporary context of social and economic inequalities and prejudice. Moreover, the problem seems to have been framed in the context of culture – thus, the focus in the DRE strategy on developing a culturally competent workforce. Fernando (2003) argues that a focus on culture can in itself be racist and therefore has to be examined in this context.

Rather, to understand the reasons why these inequalities persist we need to examine and analyse how the discourses of 'race' and mental illness intersect.

Discourses of 'race'

As mentioned earlier, one enters a contested area of knowledge when constructs of 'race' and mental illness are linked. Most authors propose that a key to understanding issues of 'race', culture and ethnicity is to be clear about how these are defined. I would argue differently. Following the lead of Cooper *et al* (2005), 'race' and ethnicity should be viewed as social constructions that will have different individual and societal meanings depending on the context in which they are applied. An important issue to consider is the meanings that are attached to 'race' and its subcomponents of ethnicity, culture and racism. More importantly, it has to be acknowledged that these constructs carry what Knowles (1999) terms 'the edifice of negative social meanings'. One can therefore not assume that all black people will assign similar meanings and values to being cast in the role of 'other' and, by implication, inferior. 'Race' also constitutes only one dimension of black identities – albeit an important one for black people: it intersects with other social divisions such as age, class, gender and sexuality.

Another issue to consider is the impact of racial disadvantage and discrimination on individuals, their families and communities. Patel and Fatimilehin (1999) suggested that the impact of racism is psychological, social and material. The effects of these are likely to be detrimental to mental health, but it has to be borne in mind that for some it may be minimal, while for others it may be of great significance to their emotional well-being. The effects of racism on the individual may have wider impacts on families and communities (McKenzie, 2002). The impact of racism therefore has to be analysed in the context of histories of migration, histories of alienation, the subordination that resonates for these groups, and the way in which these groups have been stigmatised and continue to be stigmatised in society today.

Discourses of mental illness

There are many competing discourses and perspectives on what constitutes mental illness. Bracken and Thomas (2005) argue that our knowledge of mental illness and distress is indeterminate and new ways of thinking about mental illness are constantly emerging (for a more detailed analysis and critique of the discourses on madness see Bracken & Thomas, 2005; Coppock & Hopton, 2000; Fernando, 2003). Coppock and Hopton (2000) suggest that there is ample evidence to show that mental illness is affected by social and political circumstances. Regardless of the perspective or approach that is taken to understand mental illness, it has to be acknowledged that when a person is assigned a label of mental illness they take on an identity that is stigmatised and valued negatively (Johnstone, 2001; Fernando, 2006; Knowles, 1999). Mental illness can be deeply dehumanising and alienating. It is generally regarded with anxiety and fear and leads to rejection and exclusion. A report by the Social Exclusion Unit (2004) found that people with mental health problems are among the most disadvantaged and socially excluded groups in society.

Power of mental health institutions

Psychiatry is the only branch of medicine that has legal powers to forcibly treat, restrain and control individuals. Mental health professionals have the power to name and rename emotional distress. Pilgrim (2005) posits that racial biases mean black people are disproportionately dealt with by specialist mental health services and, as these services are characterised by coercive practices, one could construe this as structural disadvantage.

'Blackness' and 'madness'

The stereotype of 'big, black and dangerous' has been fixed in the popular consciousness by sensationalist media coverage of the case of Christopher Clunis – a black man who had a diagnosis of schizophrenia, who randomly killed a stranger to him, Jonathan Zito, in a London underground station in 1992. Keating *et al* (2002) have demonstrated that such stereotypical views of black people, racism, cultural ignorance, stigma and anxiety associated with mental illness often combine to influence the way in which mental health services assess and respond to the needs of BME communities.

The issue for black people is two-fold. In life generally, they have to continually negotiate their interactions in the context of being measured against how they fit the norm; in mental health, they have to cope with/manage public (mis)conceptions about black people that have also become embedded in mental health practices.

What is clear from the above is that there are at least three factors that underpin black people's experiences of the mental health system: one, how black people are treated in society; two, how people with mental health problems are treated in society, and three, the power of institutions to control and coerce people with mental health problems. Black people's experiences in society have an impact on their mental and emotional well-being; these experiences in turn influence how they experience and perceive mental health services, and their position (historical and contemporary) in society affects how they are treated in mental health services. These factors interact to produce what Trivedi (2002) terms 'a spiral of oppression'. The challenge for mental health professionals is to break this spiral.

Responding positively

Engaging with and reflecting on inequality, discrimination and oppression that arise from social divisions in society is deeply challenging. It is an invitation to examine who we are: our experiences of advantage and disadvantage, power and powerlessness, inclusion and exclusion (Williams & Keating, 2005). Practitioners need to make connections between a person's lived experience, their behaviour and their distress. This means incorporating their experiences and viewpoints in an assessment of their situation. It also involves sharing and acknowledging as meaningful the everyday activities of life. Practitioners are required to document the details of people's lives. A significant aspect of understanding lived experience is to identify sources of oppression and tease out the intersections of 'race', ethnicity, culture, age, class, gender, religion and sexuality.

Some practical steps that can be taken when working with individuals from BME communities include:

- help people to find their way back to meaningful existence, meaningful relationships, meaningful connections, restored identity

- acknowledge the struggle of black people to have their voices heard and validated

- work hard against reinforcing racism and help people come to terms with damaging and negative experiences.

Eradicating the disparities in mental health treatment and outcomes for black people requires change in individual practices, but this can only be successful if supported by changes at the organisational level. Efforts to improve mental and emotional well-being for BME communities should be anchored in an understanding of history, broader societal conditions and contexts, and black people's lived experiences: not just their experiences of racism, but also how they have survived in the face of multiple adversities.

References

Bhui K, McKenzie K, Gill P (2004) Delivering mental health services for a diverse society. *British Medical Journal* **329** 363-364.

Bracken PJ, Greenslade L, Griffen B *et al* (1998) Mental health and ethnicity: an Irish dimension. *British Journal of Psychiatry* **172** 103-105.

Bracken P, Thomas P (2005) *Postpsychiatry: mental health in a postmodern world.* Oxford: Oxford University Press.

Cooper L, Beach MC, Johnson RL *et al* (2005) Delving below the surface: understanding how race and ethnicity influence relationships in health care. *Journal of General Internal Medicine* **21** (s21) 27.

Coppock V, Hopton J (2000) *Critical perspectives on mental health.* London: Routledge.

Department of Health (1999) *National service framework for mental health: modern standards and service models.* London: Department of Health.

Department of Health (2003) *Delivering race equality: a framework for action. Consultation document.* London: Department of Health.

Department of Health (2005) *Delivering race equality in mental health care: an action plan for reform inside and outside services and the government's response to the independent inquiry into the death of David Bennett.* London: Department of Health.

Fernando S (2003) *Cultural diversity, mental health and psychiatry: the struggle against racism.* Hove: Brunner-Routledge.

Fernando S (2006) Stigma, racism and power. *Ethnic Network Journal* **1** (1) 24-28.

Gilvarry CM, Walsh E, Samele C *et al* (1999) Life events, ethnicity and perceptions of discrimination in patients with severe mental illness. *Social Psychiatry and Psychiatric Epidemiology* **34** (11) 600-608.

Healthcare Commission (2005) *Count me in: results of a national census of inpatients in mental health hospitals and facilities in England and Wales.* London: Healthcare Commission.

Johnstone M (2001) Stigma, social justice and the rights of the mentally ill: challenging the status quo. *Australian and New Zealand Journal of Mental Health and Nursing* **10** 200-209.

Keating F, Robertson D (2004) Fear, black people and mental illness: a vicious circle? *Health and Social Care in the Community* **12** (5) 439–447.

Keating F, Robertson D, Francis F *et al* (2002) *Breaking the circles of fear: a review of the relationship between mental health services and African and Caribbean communities.* London: Sainsbury Centre for Mental Health.

Knowles C (1999) Race, identities and lives. *The Sociological Review* **47** (1) 110-135.

McKenzie K (2002) Understanding racism in mental health. In: Bhui K (ed) *Racism and mental health: prejudice and suffering.* London: Jessica Kingsley Publishers.

Morgan C, Mallett R, Hutchinson G *et al* (2004) Negative pathways to psychiatric care and ethnicity: the bridge between social science and psychiatry. *Social Science and Medicine* **58** 739-752.

Norfolk, Suffolk and Cambridgeshire Strategic Health Authority (2003) *Independent inquiry into the death of David Bennett.* Norfolk: Cambridgeshire Strategic Health Authority.

Patel N, Fatimilehin I (1999) Racism and mental health. In: Newnes C, Holmes G, Dunn C (eds) *This is madness: a critical look at psychiatry and the future of mental health services.* Ross-on-Wye: PCCS Books.

Pilgrim D (2005) *Key concepts in mental health.* London: Sage Publications.

Rogers A, Pilgrim D (2003) *Mental health and inequality.* Basingstoke: Palgrave MacMillan.

Social Exclusion Unit (2004) *Mental health and social exclusion.* London: ODPM.

Trivedi P (2002) Racism, social exclusion and mental health: a black service user's perspective. In: Bhui K (ed) *Racism and mental health: prejudice and suffering.* London: Jessica Kingsley Publishers.

White A (2002) *Social focus in brief: ethnicity.* London: Office for National Statistics.

Williams J, Keating F (2005) Social inequalities and mental health. In: Bell A, Lindley P (eds) *Beyond the water towers: the unfinished revolution in mental health services 1985–2005.* London: Sainsbury Centre for Mental Health.

Chapter 5
Challenging discrimination against people with mental health problems

Graham Thornicroft

People always said that Rachel was very clever. For some, this made it more difficult to understand her when she began to develop mental health problems: 'When I was ill at university, they really didn't know what to do about it.' Her parents also struggled to understand her changing behaviour: 'My mother, she gets over-anxious which is very debilitating. She just worries, worries, worries, which just exacerbates the whole thing. And my dad used to say, "You ought to pull yourself together".' Initially her doctors did not tell her the diagnosis. Not knowing what her condition was, she was reluctant to continue to take medication. 'So I went to my GP, and he said it's very dangerous to come off the drugs. So I came off the drugs and got psychotic again and that's when I lost another two jobs.' Eventually one of her doctors did disclose her diagnosis. 'I went to see a psychiatrist and he said, "Do you think you're causing plane crashes and that the television is talking to you?" I said yes, yes, yes, yes, yes, and he said, "Well, you're schizophrenic." It was so enormously helpful to think: (a) this was something diagnosable and (b) there are self-help groups. I don't think I've lost a job since then, partly because I was medicated. At least it was something that you thought people understood.'

Rachel's mental illness has affected many aspects of her life. Finding boyfriends has been hard. 'I manage my illness. It's something I deal with. It's very much a part of me. It's not something I go on about. Nice men are afraid of upsetting you and are a bit wary, which is extremely frustrating. I would rather they thought, "Well you're managing this and it's your choice".'

She has suffered financially from her condition: for example, she has to pay higher premiums for insurance. 'My endowment policy from my mortgage is a higher rate. I pay more because I'm ill. I think it's 15-20% more. I disclosed my condition because otherwise you end up not being covered at all.' Travel insurance is also a continuing problem: 'If I broke a leg I would be covered, but not for a previously existing condition.'

Rachel is sure that discrimination against her at work has been worse than any other consequence of her mental illness. Her dilemmas started in not knowing whether to disclose her medical history when applying for jobs. 'There is a whole issue about whether you tell people or not. If you tell people, they turn you down at interview unless its public sector, when they have a quota. Sometimes they say "We won't touch that". In [my last] job, if I had said about my mental illness I might not have got the job. I would say disclose and discuss it, but knowing that you might not get the job because of it. It's horrible. That's the worst thing for everybody.'

Despite this, Rachel has successfully found many jobs, but she feels she was not always treated fairly when she was unwell – although, looking back, she thinks her employers sometimes had good reasons to sack her when she was unwell. 'I had 20 jobs in five years, and I was being sacked because I really wasn't very well. For [my last] job, they should have had a proper chat with me rather than just sack me. But at that point I went off my medication and from their point of view I just wasn't doing the job properly. So I didn't complain, but I think it could have been handled differently.'

She now works where her personal experience of mental illness is positively valued. 'In my current job it was explicitly stated in the advertisements that knowledge of mental health was an advantage.' Still, she feels that her promotion prospects are damaged by declaring that she has a mental illness. 'If you put that you are in a wheelchair it's fine, but for mental illness there are subtle ways that you are treated differently. You can't put your finger on it really. I applied for a job on a government advisory committee, and I didn't get it. You can't help feeling that they would rather have someone in a wheelchair, or blind people or deaf people. They don't know quite where to pigeonhole you.'

Rachel has developed her own ways of coping with her problems. 'I have learned mechanisms of coping with other people in the office, and I don't go around telling other people usually, and people don't notice so it must be all right. You learn to accommodate things. I'm articulate, and you get a sort of alley-cat attitude and instinct about situations and about sensing things. I've made a huge effort with friends and I have loads of friends. Because interpersonal relationships are difficult when you are ill I have really concentrated on it, and now it's one of my major skills, I think. You overcompensate in a way.'

She says she has learned by hard experience how ignorant most people – even the educated middle classes – are about mental illness. 'Everybody knows very little about it. Because most of the publicity is negative, about violence and so on. There's no information for people, is there? Also they don't like talking about it, and half of them are worried they've got a little bit of something themselves.'

Beyond stigma

Unfortunately, Rachel's experiences are far from uncommon. In fact, there is widespread evidence that many people with mental illness suffer disadvantage and discrimination in many aspects of their lives – and that this phenomenon is global: there is no country, society or culture in which people with mental illness are considered to have the same value and to be as acceptable as people who do not have mental illness. Moreover, mental illness carries a far greater stigma than any other condition (Lai *et al*, 2001; Lee *et al*, 2005; Sartorius & Schulze, 2005).

However, while the concept of stigma is necessary to develop an understanding of experiences of social exclusion, it does not usefully inform the practical steps that need to be taken to promote social inclusion.

In this context stigma can be seen as the conjunction of three problems (Thornicroft, 2006a; 2006b):

- problem of ignorance = ignorance
- problem of attitudes   = prejudice
- problem of behaviour = discrimination.

Repeated surveys show that exclusion from the employment market is experienced as one of worst effects of stigma (Read & Baker, 1996; Becker *et al*, 1996). A large study in Germany (Schulze & Angermeyer, 2003), for example, found that stigma was experienced most powerfully in relation to:

- interpersonal interactions
- structural discrimination
- public images of mental illness
- access to meaningful social roles, especially at work.

Employment offers social networks, a route out of poverty, and a source of social status in market economies. Over time, unemployment often leads to a loss of confidence, and a sense of being without any social value.

> 'I lost my job. I was unwell. I was having a lot of difficulties. I couldn't tolerate being sacked again. I've given up. Once bitten, twice shy.' (Kim)

Work can promote good mental health. It offers opportunities for control and using skills, externally generated goals, variety, environmental clarity, money, physical security, interpersonal contact, and a valued social position (Warr, 1987).

> 'This is my workplace. This is where I earn my definition, the place that tells me what I am.' (Galloway, 1991)

Yet the simple fact is that a diagnosis of mental illness is one of the most powerful explanations for exclusion from the workforce (Warner, 2004). The employment rate for the whole adult population is about 75%; for people with physical health problems it is about 65%, but only some 20% of people with more severe mental health problems are employed (SEU, 2004). Only half of people with more common types of mental illness, such as depression, are competitively employed (Meltzer *et al*, 1995). Yet people with mental disorders have the highest 'want to work' rate: overall, 52% of the disabled people interviewed in one survey wanted to find a job; among people with 'mental illness, phobias and panics' this figure rose to 86% (Stanley & Maxwell, 2004).

This gap may be getting worse: employment rates for people with a diagnosis of schizophrenia, for example, seem to have fallen during the last 50 years in many economically developed countries (Marwaha & Johnson, 2004). Indeed, the need for a meaningful link to society through work may be even greater for some people with mental illness if they experience isolation or exclusion in other areas of their lives (Repper & Perkins, 2003).

'I have never suffered from such cruelty because when applying for jobs I never admitted to my own depression. If I had, I would never have stood a chance. People are frightened about anything to do with mental illness, they just do not understand the malady.' (David)

Why is finding and keeping a job so difficult for so many people with a diagnosis of mental illness? One explanation is that employers discriminate against applicants who declare a history of psychiatric treatment. One study, involving human resource officers, found that the mention of a mental illness significantly reduced applicants' chances of employment, but this was not the case where an applicant disclosed a diagnosis of diabetes (Glozier, 1998). Moreover, this differential treatment was based on perceptions of potential poor work performance, rather than expectations of absenteeism.

'I haven't applied for any jobs since I've become ill. To stop me applying is a part of the anxieties and the things that I have as part of the syndrome of mine and is just lack of confidence, you know… I don't really have that much ambitious goals – just get a decent job and, you know, a decent reasonable living. That's what I wanted to do. But I haven't been able to do that yet because of my illness so far. But I feel much better now I'm getting ready to get back to employment.' (Leroy)

Problems with concentration and memory can harm a person's chances of getting or keeping a job, and it is likely that some people will need both occupational support to find jobs and psychological treatment to help them with their cognitive problems. A major dilemma faced by people with a history of psychiatric treatment is whether to disclose this when applying for a job. There are good reasons to believe that mentioning this will reduce the likelihood of success. On the other hand, failure to disclose will mean that the person is not able to ask for modifications to the job to make it more manageable (often called 'reasonable adjustments' or 'reasonable accommodations') (Corrigan, 2004; Repper & Perkins, 2003).

'An employer would see my diagnosis of schizophrenia as a disadvantage, and so I would be reluctant even to apply for a job. I would expect myself to be in a more disadvantaged position than a normal person.' (Raj)

There is no easy solution to this dilemma. One approach is to make a balance sheet of the advantages and disadvantages of disclosing a history of mental illness, and to use this in making a decision (Corrigan & Lundin, 2001).

Paradoxically, there is evidence that mental health services may be especially unforgiving when their own staff suffer from mental illness. In many countries the health and social services are major players in the labour market: the NHS in the UK, for example, is the largest employer in Europe. Yet healthcare organisations are particularly poor both at keeping staff who become mentally ill and at taking on new staff who have a history of mental illness. One leading psychologist in England puts it like this:

'I've encountered all those hushed conversations along the lines of, "Is she really all right? Is she really able to work?" ... particularly from other clinical psychologists, who have difficulties with a high-profile member of their own profession being open about having mental health problems.'

There is one way to jump-start this process: to encourage health and social care agencies to see the experience of mental illness as a positive attribute when hiring staff. They can do this by making it clear that a personal knowledge of mental illness – for example, as a consumer or a carer – is seen as a positive advantage for qualified applicants. However this is done, it means reversing the common tendency in health and social services to see workers as either healthy and strong donors of care, or as weak and vulnerable recipients.

For some people with mental illness, modifications may need to be made at work to accommodate their personal needs – what are known as 'reasonable adjustments' in the Disability Discrimination Act (DDA). Practically speaking, what does this mean in the workplace? One of the challenges here is that, while employers can understand the need for an entrance ramp for people in wheelchairs, often they do not know how to apply this concept to people with mental illnesses. Such support may assume different forms, such as:

- for people with concentration problems, having a quieter work station with fewer distractions, rather than a noisy, open-plan office, and a rest area for breaks

- more, or more frequent, supervision than usual, to give feedback and guidance on job performance

- allowing a person to use headphones to block out distracting noise

- flexibility in work hours so that they can attend their healthcare appointments, or work when not impaired by medication

- a buddy/mentor scheme to provide on-site orientation and assistance

- clear person specifications, job descriptions and task assignments to assist people who find ambiguity or uncertainty hard to cope with

- for people likely to become unwell for prolonged periods, it may be necessary to make contract modifications to specifically allow whatever sickness leave they need

- a more gradual induction phase – for example, with more time to complete tasks for those who return to work after a prolonged absence, or who may have some cognitive impairment

- improved disability awareness in the workplace, to reduce stigma and to underpin all other accommodations

- reallocation of marginal job functions that are disturbing to an individual

- allowing use of accrued paid and unpaid leave for periods of illness.

It can be argued that these provisions should be made available to everyone, not only to those people who have a mental health problem. Also, the adjustments needed by an individual may well change over time and need to be reviewed regularly. Clear arrangements on confidentiality are necessary: if a job applicant does disclose having a mental illness and changes are made to their working arrangements, who needs to know this? In particular, for people working in the same organisation in which they are treated for their mental illness, specific safeguards are needed to ensure that the confidentiality of clinical information is safeguarded.

It is time to stop thinking that stigma is somehow inevitable and unchangeable and instead to regard inclusion in the job market as one of the most important ways in which we can combat discrimination against people with mental illness. The primary remedy is clear: to apply disability discrimination laws equally for people with physical and mental illness related disabilities. But this is much more than just a question of legal procedure. Winning full parity in how legal entitlements are put into practice needs to be seen as part of a wider civil rights movement by people with mental illness.

Graham Thornicroft's book Shunned: discrimination against people with mental illness *is published by Oxford University Press.*

References

Becker DR, Drake RE, Farabaugh A *et al* (1996) Job preferences of clients with severe psychiatric disorders participating in supported employment programs. *Psychiatric Services* **47** (11) 1223-1226.

Corrigan PW (2004) *On the stigma of mental illness: practical strategies for research and social change*. Washington, DC: American Psychological Association.

Corrigan P, Lundin R (2001) *Don't call me nuts*. Tinley Par, Illinois: Recovery Press.

Galloway J (1991) *The trick is to keep breathing*. London: Minerva.

Glozier N (1998) Workplace effects of the stigmatization of depression. *Journal of Occupational and Environmental Medicine* **40** (9) 793-800.

Lai YM, Hong CP, Chee CY (2001) Stigma of mental illness. *Singapore Medical Journal* **42** (3) 111-114.

Lee S, Lee MT, Chiu MY *et al* (2005) Experience of social stigma by people with schizophrenia in Hong Kong. *British Journal of Psychiatry* **186** 153-157.

Marwaha S, Johnson S (2004) Schizophrenia and employment: a review. *Social Psychiatry and Psychiatric Epidemiology* **39** (5) 337-349.

Meltzer H, Gill B, Pettierew M *et al* (1995) *OPCS surveys of psychiatric morbidity in Great Britain. Report 3: Economic activity and social functioning of adults with psychiatric disorders*. London: HMSO.

Read J, Baker S (1996) *Not just sticks and stones: a survey of the stigma, taboos and discrimination experienced by people with mental health problems*. London: Mind.

Repper J, Perkins R (2003) *Social inclusion and recovery*. Edinburgh: Bailliere Tindall.

Sartorius N, Schulze H (2005) *Reducing the stigma of mental illness: a report from a global programme of the World Psychiatric Association*. Cambridge: Cambridge University Press.

Schulze B, Angermeyer MC (2003) Subjective experiences of stigma: a focus group study of schizophrenic patients, their relatives and mental health professionals. *Social Science and Medicine* **5** (2) 299-312.

Social Exclusion Unit (2004) *Mental health and social exclusion*. London: Office of the Deputy Prime Minister.

Stanley K, Maxwell D (2004) *Fit for purpose?* London: ippr.

Thornicroft G (2006a) *Actions speak louder: tackling discrimination against people with mental illness*. London: Mental Health Foundation.

Thornicroft G (2006b) *Shunned: discrimination against people with mental illness*. Oxford: Oxford University Press.

Warner R (2004) *Recovery from schizophrenia: psychiatry and political economy (3rd edition)*. Hove: Brunner-Routledge.

Warr P (1987) *Work, unemployment and mental health*. Oxford: Oxford University Press.

Chapter 6
Women's mental health and recovery

Jeanette Copperman and Fiona Hill

Research has repeatedly shown that women's mental health is not just a matter of individual pathology but is intimately connected to life experiences, and in particular to social inequalities that impact on women's life chances. However, mainstream mental health services continue to be dominated by an individualised and medicalised approach to mental distress that takes little account of these wider issues (Barnes *et al*, 2002; Williams *et al*, 2001a; Brown and Harris, 1978). In this chapter we are going to give an overview of what is known about women's mental health, the factors that influence women's mental well-being, and current government policy on meeting women's mental health needs. We will also highlight the main issues that women who use services have identified as important, and show how their needs can be met through a recovery-oriented, person-centred approach.

Women's mental health

Although considerable progress has been made over the last 30 years, women still occupy a socially unequal position in our society. Women are restricted in their access to economic, social and political power, to well-paid work, and in the roles that they are able to play (EOC, 2006). Overall, women's gross income is still only 49% of men's. Women are also subject to violence and abuse more frequently than men, throughout their lives, whether it is physical and sexual abuse in childhood or rape, domestic violence or elder abuse as adults. It is estimated that one in four women will experience domestic violence at some point in their life, and in a third of cases the violence will start or get worse during pregnancy (Domestic Violence Data Source, 2002). Many women receiving mental health services report previous experience of violence and abuse (Bryer *et al*, 1987; Harris & Landis, 1997). It has been estimated that more than a half of all women receiving treatment in mental health services have experienced psychical or sexual abuse in childhood (Jacobson, 1989).

In addition to experience of violence, in almost every instance the socio-economic and psychological factors known to affect mental health impact on women more severely than men.

■ Poverty. Women – and lone parent and older women in particular – are more likely than men to live in poverty. Two thirds of adults living in the poorest households and two thirds of those dependent on benefits are women.

■ Employment. Nearly twice as many women (30%) than men (16%) of working age do not have a job, and only 35% of women are in full-time paid employment. The majority are in part-time, low-paid work. Unemployment is linked with mental health problems.

■ Carer responsibilities. Women do most of the caring for children and other family dependents, even if they also work.

■ Life events. Experiences such as loss or bereavement are associated with depression; feeling threatened and unsafe is associated with anxiety.

■ Social isolation. Women are more vulnerable to social isolation than men, for all the socio-economic reasons cited above, and because of their longer life expectancy and the fact that they are less free than men to go out and more dependent on public transport when they do. Social isolation is known to affect mental health. (Department of Health, 2003)

Particular groups of women may be more vulnerable to mental ill health: women who are mothers or have other caring responsibilities, older women, women from black and minority ethnic groups, lesbian and bisexual women, transsexual women, women involved in the sex trade, and women offenders. It is known that women serving a prison sentence are twice as likely as men to have received treatment for mental health problems in the preceding 12 months, and are more likely than male prisoners to have a history of self-harm. Women with learning disabilities, like all people with learning disabilities, have higher rates of mental ill health, and are in addition very vulnerable to physical, sexual and emotional abuse. Women who misuse drugs or alcohol are another major at-risk group, and less likely than men to have their difficulties diagnosed and to receive help, partly because of the attached stigma. Fear of losing their children may also deter women from seeking help.

Substantial research evidence also shows that concepts of mental health and illness are constructed in a gendered way: that the distribution of diagnoses differs according to gender, and that particular factors in women's lives contribute to the experience of mental health problems (Barnes *et al*, 2002; Pilgrim & Rogers, 2003; Prior, 1999). For example, borderline personality disorder is a diagnosis given almost exclusively to women, and many women with this diagnosis have a history of sexual abuse and self-harm (Shaw, 2005; Harris & Landis, 1997; Bryer *et al*, 1987). Studies have also shown that mental health practitioners have different expectations of what it is to be mentally 'healthy' for men and women (Broverman *et al*, 1970). In the study by Broverman and colleagues, the mature, mentally healthy individual was seen as typically male; a woman's normal mental state was seen as passive, emotional and dependent. There are numerous reports that mental health workers can be reluctant to work with women users, and that they use stigmatising language to describe female patients (Williams *et al*, 2001b).

Psychiatric injustice

Inequality, as well as determining access to money, status and power, can sustain processes that hide injustice and discrimination, and create opportunities for serious abuses of power (Williams, 2005). Williams and Keating argue that mainstream psychiatric services perpetuate practices that can mask and reinforce abuse, and this is significant for women's mental health (Williams & Keating, 2000).

The lack of safety for women using mental health services is an example of this. Women may be harassed, sexually assaulted and even raped on NHS psychiatric wards and in mental health day services (NPSA, 2006). The Department of Health introduced a policy in 2002 that all wards should provide women-only sleeping and bathroom areas. However, while 99% of mental health trusts claim to be compliant with this guidance, many women still report being admitted to mixed wards (Mind, 2004); in some cases the women's areas are separated by only a curtain or partition, and there are reports that male staff and patients do not respect the women-only areas (DUG, 2006).

The inquiry into the sexual abuse of more than 70 female patients over a 40-year period by two senior consultants, William Kerr and Michael Haslam, strongly criticised an NHS culture that refused to believe the women when they complained, and failed to follow up reports when they were made (HM Government, 2005). The inquiry described this as a 'moral failing at the heart of the NHS' and questioned whether women would be any more likely to be believed today. Women admitted under section to psychiatric wards are not infrequently exposed to the same kinds of verbal abuse and actual assault that brought them into contact with the mental health services in the first place. Moreover, the degradation and physical restraint associated with forced treatment have been identified as potentially retraumatising and revictimising for women who have already experienced trauma and abuse (Grobe, 1995; Copperman & McNamara, 1999).

Mental health policy

Mental health services have traditionally been slow to acknowledge these issues. The main framework for women's mental health service provision today is the 2003 Department of Health implementation guide Mainstreaming Gender and Women's Mental Health (Department of Health, 2003). The guidance is based on a consultation conducted in 2002 (Department of Health, 2002) that drew together the evidence about women's mental health, risk factors and treatment needs and preferences, highlighted good practice examples and made recommendations for action. The main recommendations in the guidance are outlined in *Table 1*.

Table 1: Mainstreaming gender and women's mental health

> ■ Individual assessment and care planning (ie. the Care Programme Approach) must recognise the broader context of women's lives: eg. experience of violence and abuse, caring responsibilities, cultural needs, safe housing and employment/training/education needs, respite or crisis support, and cultural needs.

> ■ Women should have access to a range of psychological, complementary and creative therapies.

> ■ Primary care services should be more responsive to women's specific mental health needs, including early identification of depression and post-natal depression, self-harm and alcohol and substance misuse; sensitivity to women's possible history of violence and abuse, including domestic violence; awareness of the dangers of long-term prescribing of benzodiazepines, anti-psychotic and anti-depressant medication, and referral to relevant community support services.

> ■ PCTs should ensure provision of women-only day services, run by women staff.

> ■ Women should have access to a range of safe and supported housing, whether or not they have children.

> ■ Women should have the choice to be admitted to a mixed ward or to a self-contained women-only ward or unit, and these should be available in every acute inpatient unit.

> ■ Women-only crisis houses should be established as an alternative to acute inpatient admission and respite care.

> ■ Community-based mental health teams (assertive outreach, crisis resolution, home treatment and early intervention) should ensure they are gender-sensitive, and in particular support women with children who may fear losing them, and ensure women are offered the choice, wherever possible, of a female care worker.

To take forward the guidance, each trust and PCT was advised to appoint a senior lead officer and establish a multi-agency forum and a local women's service user group. However, there was no ring-fenced money for implementation attached to the recommendations. Nor were the standards in the guidance included in trusts' annual performance rating targets, other than the provision of separate women's wards, which was subsequently interpreted to mean simply separate sleeping areas and bathroom facilities within mixed wards. More recent commissioning guidance on day service provision for women (Department of Health, 2006) suggests that PCTs draw on existing community initiatives and, in line with a refocus in day service provision across the board, move away from buildings-based services towards supported involvement in mainstream activities. It suggests, for example, that support workers could 'facilitate access to community activities for women', or provide creche facilities to enable them to attend mainstream leisure or education opportunities, or offer shopping or befriending services, in particular for older or disabled women.

What women say

In 2005 Brent Mental Health User Group (BUG) carried out a survey on behalf of the mental health local implementation team (LIT) to find out what women using mental health services in the borough felt about these services, and what they wanted from them in the future (BUG, 2006). The survey was based on the key areas highlighted in the Mainstreaming Gender consultation and the Department of Health implementation guidance.

The survey was user-led and user-run. A total of 73 women of a range of ages were interviewed. They included women from black and minority ethnic communities, lesbians and women with physical disabilities. What they said reflects both the conclusions in Mainstreaming Gender and other research (Barnes *et al*, 2002; Williams *et al*, 2001a).

Most of the women were very clear about where their distress came from. Of the 60 women who answered this question, 35 said their use of services was linked to their experiences of violence – including domestic violence – or harassment or discrimination:

> *'They see everything as symptoms and do not analyse that you are as you are because of life events, not through psychotic illness etc.'*

A significant number (49) felt their distress was linked to relationships, or lack of them. Some related their use of services to their experiences as children, and 20 said their role as a carer had led to their mental distress. Social issues such as housing (13 women), stress at work and work–life balance (12 women), and lack of money and lack of help at home (21) were also mentioned.

Half of the women felt professionals did not understand the reasons for their distress, including eight of the 23 Asian women. However, half did, with some saying it depended on the individual practitioner. While just over half said mental health professionals did help them deal with their feelings and distressed behaviours, many others disagreed, with only nine of the 23 Asian women and two of the seven lesbian women feeling that mental health practitioners were helpful:

> *'Doctor never gives me enough time to explain. I would like them to give me more time and really listen to me.'*

Also, the number of women who found mental health professionals helpful seemed to decrease with age: only 12 of the 33 women aged 45 and over and five of the 14 women aged 55 and over agreed that mental health professionals were helpful.

The women felt that staff were not confident about working with their experiences of abuse or violence, despite this being something women wanted. They said their different roles – as mothers, for example – were not taken into account in care planning (CPA). A number of women talked about either losing their children as a result of their distress or not being able to have contact with their children if they were in hospital. They also said they were not offered the choice of a female keyworker or psychiatrist, even where this was important to them because of their culture or sexuality. Comments indicated that, often, staff did not know how to create a culture that would make women-only space and activities possible and safe for women.

Very few of the women were using women-only community groups or groups providing specialist services to black and minority ethnic communities, people with disabilities, or other minority groups. Asked what they liked about services provided to women only, 14 out of 18 said they felt safer and 'found it easier to talk to women'; 13 said they felt more comfortable, and nine said it was easier to work in a group with women.

Some women said they had felt safe in hospital, but a number talked about feeling unsafe and that they couldn't use the women's spaces on wards because of both staff members' and male service users' behaviour. They also said that male staff generally did not respect women's spaces or ask for permission before going into a woman's room, if she was lucky enough to have one. The separate bathroom and toilet facilities were frequently disregarded:

'When given the choice of sleeping in the women-only section I felt safer from past experience. The male patients hassled the female patients for sex and went into the female dormitories.'

What women want

The Brent women wanted the staff to be approachable and friendly, understanding, respectful and patient. They wanted to be listened to when they tried to talk about their distress and where it comes from; they wanted staff to talk to them about their medication, how it works and alternatives to it and the side effects of medication. They also wanted to be asked what they felt they needed, and for staff to understand their culture, and act on what they said:

'I think the most important thing of all, that staff could learn to do better, is listen to and take seriously what people like me are saying.'

The women also said they wanted staff to work with them towards recovery, and to recognise the reasons for their distress and build on their own beliefs and coping strategies. Women also wanted a choice to take part in women-only activities.

It was also clear that women wanted staff to use different approaches to dealing with their distress and not just focus on medication. Access to talking treatments was highlighted.

'Re medication, some issues are discussed like gaining weight, but no discussion about the differences in the way dosages affect men and women. Ways I have of coping were only discussed in relation to drugs.'

Recovery approaches

Recovery approaches take account of service users' personal experiences, their whole lives and their beliefs about the nature and sources of their distress. Recovery approaches also acknowledge and value the coping strategies people have developed to manage their mental distress, and make explicit the impact of stigma and discrimination on people's well-being (Wallcraft, 2005; Anthony, 1993). For this reason, a recovery approach provides an ideal framework for women's mental health care.

Repper and Perkins (2003) identify three core components to recovery-oriented practice:

- developing hope-inspiring relationships
- facilitating understanding, acceptance and taking back control
- helping people to access the roles, relationships and activities that are important to them.

Adopting a recovery-oriented approach enables practitioners to move away from a focus on people's problems and deficits (the 'broken brain' approach). Instead the focus is on people's strengths and abilities, and the person is fully involved in deciding their own goals and how they attain them.

At national level, values-based, recovery-oriented practices are now considered to provide the basis for good practice in mental health (NIMHE, 2004). BUG has incorporated three key elements of these in a training programme for mental health support workers, as follows.

Reframing

Reframing is a practical tool to assist mental health workers to turn negative beliefs about people who use services into positive opportunities to find ways to work with them. So, for example, labels often used to describe women with mental health problems include 'manipulative', 'attention-seeking', and 'boundary-less'. Reframed, manipulative becomes 'resourceful', attention-seeking becomes 'knowing and saying what you need', and boundary-less becomes 'trying to form relationships'.

By removing the label, reframing also allows workers to see the individual, get to know her and work with her strengths.

A strengths-based approach

In the strengths-based approach the focus is on women's strengths and abilities, not deficits and problems, and helping women to use them to deal with difficulties. Too often women with mental health problems come to believe that their mental ill health defines them; they feel infantilised by the mental health system and lose confidence in their own abilities to manage their lives. Using a strengths-based approach practitioners draw on the skills and abilities women have in other areas of their lives, such as their parenting skills, and help them think how these could be applied in other contexts. A practical example of using reframing linked with a strengths-based approach might be a woman who is highly sociable and chatty and wants to develop relationships. The staff see her as lacking boundaries. Reframed, her chattiness and social skills might make her a good befriender, or she might like to work with people in a user-run café. Women have often developed coping strategies to deal with their life experiences. Staff can work with a woman to help her identify and use these strengths in managing her distress and moving forward.

Positive risk-taking

Mental health services have increasingly adopted defensive practice, partly through fear of blame if something goes wrong. Staff therefore do not encourage women to take risks by setting new goals, beyond the confines imposed on their lives and aspirations by their mental distress. Positive risk-taking is about considering with women what they want to achieve, however simple or apparently small – it could be going back to work; it could be simply getting out of the house every day – and helping them map out manageable steps towards it. It includes considering what social supports the woman already has, and what she might need to enable her to take on new challenges; what has helped in the past, and what contingency plans she might want to put in place.

Self-harm is often cited by practitioners as a real challenge when working with women who use mental health services (Williams, 2001b). Positive risk-taking can offer a new approach. For many women, self-harm is in fact a coping strategy, not an attempt at suicide. Rather than telling a woman not to self-harm, a practitioner might work with her to enable her to do so safely, to look after herself, to find other ways of releasing emotions (MHF, 1997; 2006; Arnold, 1998; Pembroke, 2006a; 2006b).

BUG has produced a very simple tool to help women 'design their own lives'. This is a set of illustrated A5 cards covering various aspects of women's lives such as learning new skills, using self-help groups, having pets, doing exercise, dealing with housing issues, socialising etc, that can be used to enable women to think more creatively about what they want from their lives.

Conclusion

There is now a great deal of research and information about what women want from mental health services. Good national policy exists, but higher priority needs to be given to implementation of services that meet women's needs, drawing on the flexibility and innovation offered in the voluntary sector.

The Brent Mental Health User Group (BUG) survey showed that women feel mainstream mental health practitioners can be an important resource and that they would value their help and support. However it also showed that practitioners lack confidence and skills in working with women and the issues they bring, suggesting a need for training.

Staff can ensure that services do not replicate the reasons for women needing to use mental health services, by creating an environment that is both emotionally and physically safe. The Mainstreaming Gender guidance, coupled with the recovery approach, presents opportunities for services to develop a range of approaches and alternative treatments and social interventions that recognise the validity of people's own beliefs and understandings about their distress. The challenge is for mental health services to move away from focusing on chronicity towards these approaches, creating an organisational context and culture within which mental health practitioners can work creatively and effectively with women.

References

Anthony WA (1993) Recovery from mental illness: the guiding vision of the mental health service system in the 1990s. *Psychosocial Rehabilitation Journal* **16** (4) 11-23.

Arnold L (1998) Counselling people who self injure. In: Bear Z (ed) *Good practice in counselling people who have been abused.* London: Jessica Kingsley Publishers.

Barnes M, Davis A, Guru S *et al* (2002) *Women-only and women-sensitive mental health services: an expert paper.* Final report to the Department of Health. Unpublished.

Brent Mental Health User Group (2006) *Survey of women using services to deal with mental health issues.* Brent: BUG. Available from admin@brentusergroup.com or downloadable from http://kc.nimhe.org.uk

Broverman K, Broverman D, Clarkson F *et al* (1970) Sex role stereotypes and clinical judgements of mental health. *Journal of Consulting and Clinical Psychology* **34** (1) 1-7.

Brown GW, Harris T (1978) *Social origins of depression.* London: Tavistock Publications.

Bryer J, Nelson BA, Miller JB (1987) Childhood sexual and physical abuse as factors in adult psychiatric illness. *American Journal of Psychiatry* **144** (11) 1426-1431.

Copperman J, McNamara J (1999) Institutional abuse in mental health settings: survivor perspectives. In: Stanley N, Manthorpe J, Penhale B (eds) *Institutional abuse: perspectives across the life course.* London: Routledge.

Department of Health (2002) *Women's mental health: into the mainstream. Strategic development of mental health care for women.* London: Department of Health.

Department of Health (2003) *Mainstreaming gender and women's mental health: implementation guidance.* London: Department of Health.

Department of Health (2006) *Supporting women into the mainstream: commissioning women-only community day services.* London: Department of Health.

Domestic Violence Data Source (2002) *Factsheets 1-5.* www.domesticvioencedata.org/4-faqs/facts.htm

Equal Opportunities Commission (2006) *Facts about women and men in Great Britain.* Manchester: Equal Opportunities Commission.

Grobe J (1995) Hospital records. In: Grobe J (ed) *Beyond Bedlam: contemporary women psychiatric survivors speak out.* Chicago: Third Side Press.

Harris M, Landis L (1997) *Sexual abuse in the lives of women diagnosed with serious mental illness.* London: Harwood Academic.

HM Government (2005) *The Kerr/Haslam inquiry.* Cm 6640. London: The Stationery Office.

Jacobson A (1989) Physical and sexual assault histories among psychiatric outpatients. *American Journal of Psychiatry* **146** 755-758.

Mental Health Foundation (1997) *Bristol crisis service for women – training on self-harm.* Briefing no. 2. London: Mental Health Foundation.

Mental Health Foundation (2006) *Truth hurts: report of the national inquiry into self-harm among young people.* London: Mental Health Foundation.

Mind (2004) *Wardwatch: Mind's report on hospital conditions for mental health patients.* London: Mind.

NIMHE (2004) *Emerging best practices in mental health recovery.* York: NIMHE North East Development Centre.

NPSA (2006) *With safety in mind: mental health services and patient safety.* London: NPSA.

Pembroke L (2006a) Limiting the damage. *Mental Health Today* (April) 27-30.

Pembroke L (2006b) Offer us what we want. *Mental Health Today* (July/August) 16-19.

Pilgrim D, Rogers A (2003) *Mental health and inequality.* Basingstoke: Palgrave Macmillan.

Prior PM (1999) *Gender and mental health.* Basingstoke: Macmillan Press.

Repper J, Perkins R (2003) *Social inclusion and recovery.* London: Balliere Tindall.

Shaw C (2005) An activist/user perspective on challenging policy on borderline personality disorder. In: Social Perspectives Network. *Turning rhetoric into reality: sharing practice perspectives and strategies for action on women's mental health.* Study day 7. London: Social Perspectives Network.

Wallcraft J (2005) Recovery from mental breakdown. In: Tew J (ed) *Social perspectives in mental health.* London: Jessica Kingsley.

Williams J (2005) Women's mental health: taking inequality into account. In: Tew J (ed) *Social perspectives in mental heath.* London: Jessica Kingsley.

Williams J, Keating F (2000) Abuse in mental health services: some theoretical considerations. *The Journal of Adult Protection* **2** (3) 32-39.

Williams J, LeFrancois B, Copperman J (2001a) *Mental health services that work for women: survey findings.* Canterbury: Tizard Centre, University of Kent.

Williams J, Scott S, Waterhouse S (2001b) Mental health services for 'difficult' women: reflections on some recent developments. *Feminist Review* **68** (summer) 1-16.

Chapter 7
Everybody's business: mental health in older age

Ros Levenson and Catherine Jackson

The mental health of older people is a sorely neglected area. It has to be stressed that mental ill health is not an inevitable part of ageing: most older people (like most younger adults) enjoy good mental health and well-being. But there are particular mental health problems that are associated with old age – specifically, of course, dementia. Moreover, older people are more vulnerable to the stresses and psycho-social factors that are known to lead to mental health problems in anyone of any age: physical ill health and chronic pain, loss and bereavement, social isolation, poverty and loss of meaning and purpose to life. Prevalence of mental health problems in the 65+ age group is higher than in any other age group, but these factors can be tackled; the problem is, too often they aren't. Too often older people are told (or tell themselves): 'What can you expect at your age?' This chapter aims to show that older people can expect, and are entitled to, much more.

Government policy

The mental health needs of people aged 65+ are covered by standard 7 of the national service framework for older people (Department of Health, 2001). This states:

'Older people who have mental health problems have access to integrated mental health services, provided by the NHS and councils to ensure effective diagnosis, treatment and support, for them and for their carers.'

It requires NHS and local authority services to have in place jointly agreed protocols for the care and management of older people with mental health problems and plans for an integrated mental health service, including mental health promotion. It also, importantly, introduced the keystone for integrated service provision: person-centred care delivered through a single assessment process, as stated in standard 2:

'NHS and social care services treat older people as individuals and enable them to make choices about their own care. This is achieved through the single assessment process, integrated commissioning arrangements and integrated provision of services.'

Table 1: the facts

There are currently some 10.9 million people aged 65 and over in the UK. Within this 10.9 million:

- 3% will have severe and lasting depression
- 15% will have 'common mental disorders' such as depression, anxiety, panic attacks and neuroses (RCPsych, 2006).

Dementia affects one in 20 people aged 65+, and one in five people aged 80+ (RCPsych, 2006).

Prevalence of schizophrenia in later life is between 0.1% and 0.4%.

It is estimated that mental ill health affects:

- 40% of older people being treated by their GP
- 50% of older people receiving hospital treatment
- 60% of older people in residential care, of whom 40% will have depression (CSIP, 2005).

Many older people are the main carers for another older person, which of itself makes them more vulnerable to mental ill health (Singleton *et al*, 2002).

But health and social services have struggled to achieve these targets, often because of funding issues (different budgets), service boundaries (is this a health or social care issue?), and poor knowledge of mental health issues among general medical and nursing staff in hospitals. While this is not supposed to happen, older people whose mental health problems started earlier in life still find themselves passed automatically from adult mental health services to the older people's services at age 65. This can mean their care is disrupted, and they may be barred from using day services where they are settled and that are an important support in their life. Older people are frequently denied, or not offered, services available to younger people, such as psychology and counselling (Healthcare Commission, 2006).

Aware of these problems, in 2005 the Department of Health issued the policy document Securing Better Mental Health for Older Adults (Department of Health, 2005). This states clearly the principles on which health and social care services should be provided to older people:

> *'Mainstream primary care, intermediate care, hospital care, residential and other long-term care services all need to be able to accommodate the care of older people with mental health problems as these often co-exist with other problems.'*

This means all health and social care staff in any setting should have the skills at least to identify, manage initially and refer on for specialist assessment older people with mental health needs.

It also states explicitly that: '... there should be no automatic transfer of people from younger adult to older adult services at the age of 65... It should be possible for people to access appropriate components of both younger and older adult services without transferring care co-ordination responsibilities.'

Subsequently the Care Services Improvement Partnership (responsible for driving forward the implementation of the national service frameworks) issued Everybody's Business, a guide to the development of integrated mental health services for older adults (CSIP, 2005). This builds on the principles of the national service framework and of Securing Better Mental Health for Older Adults, and is today is regarded as the main policy document that should guide service development and provision.

What older people say

'Once you are a "mental patient" that is all you are allowed to be. They strip you bare of any vestiges of culture, class, beliefs, education, experience of motherhood and grandmotherhood and what you might have achieved.'

'I have never felt that my current GP has really respected my issues. He... tends to say, "What can you expect at your age?" ... I feel deeply depressed and often isolated and I truly hate it. I feel that age is a yardstick GPs use to limit me.'

'They seem to always fire drugs at people. Doctors don't seem to listen enough to what you have to say.'

'The local mental health team do not allow people over 65 to use their facilities. You are told your service is terminated and that you should attend the day centre for older people despite the fact that you may have attended the mental health day centre for many years... [This] deprives you of the company of younger people and is very upsetting.'

'Too many people are unaware of any choices and many are told that they are "unsuitable" for talking therapies.'

(Mind, 2005)

Prevention and mental health promotion

Before going on to describe areas where services are failing older people with mental health needs, it is important to repeat that much mental ill health among older people can be avoided. A Mental Health Foundation/Age Concern national inquiry into mental health and well-being in later life (MHF, 2006) identifies five key factors that affect mental health in later life:

- public attitudes (both mental health stigma and discrimination and ageism)
- staying active

- social networks
- standards of living (poverty, poor housing)
- physical health.

Black and minority ethnic people

In Bradford a Health Action Zone (a special government-funded initiative to tackle health inequalities in deprived areas) project has been set up to provide support to family carers from minority ethnic groups who care for people with dementia. The project's goal is to develop culturally appropriate dementia services by recruiting carers from minority ethnic groups. It has developed training for facilitators who then work with support groups of carers, teaching them about dementia and dementia care. The support groups also enable the carers to support each other. This has enabled carers to care for their family member and has also increased use of services by black and minority ethic people with dementia and their carers.

The inquiry panel talked to many older people, including older people from black and minority ethnic communities, about what makes for good mental well-being. What they said is no different to what anyone would say: they talked about secure and appropriate housing (accessible, for example, for people with physical disabilities, and safe), enough income to enjoy holidays and treats as well as cover basic living costs, good (or as good as possible) physical health, friends and family networks around them, and keeping active and involved in their local communities. Perhaps above all, they talked about respect: being seen as valued members of their family, and of society.

Something can be done about all these things. It means making sure public services such as leisure and sports facilities and libraries are accessible and welcoming to older people, and that public transport is available so older people can get there. It means provision of social activities and support groups for people at risk of social isolation. It also requires home care workers, social services support workers and anyone providing health and social support services to older people to be alert to these issues and to encourage older people to keep active, stay involved, take part in voluntary activities and take up new (and old) interests. It also means making sure they are getting the benefits to which they are entitled.

One recent initiative from the government's Social Exclusion Unit (2006) is applying the principles of the Sure Start programme for children and families to the needs of the most vulnerable older people in the community. In some areas there are 'one-stop' centres where vulnerable older people can get help on all these fronts.

A particular concern highlighted in the Mental Health Foundation/Age Concern inquiry report is the needs of older people from black and minority ethnic communities, whose different cultural needs may go unacknowledged, and who themselves may be experiencing the distressing effects of cultural dislocation within their own communities as their children adopt western lifestyles and attitudes. It is often (wrongly) assumed that people from BME communities 'look after their own'. There may also be specific implications for mental health in later life of the experiences of migration and lifelong racism. All communities will have culturally ingrained attitudes towards and beliefs about mental ill health that may not be helpful to the person concerned; lack of understanding about mental health problems associated with growing older (see, for example, Seabrooke & Milne's research (2004) with one south Asian community in the UK) may need to be addressed by information and education.

Everybody's Business makes the important point that older people from BME communities may not be 'hard to reach'; they may simply find services inaccessible, unwelcoming and not what they want or need. It says BME communities themselves should be involved more in saying what kind of health and social services they want, and that there should be more and better information for BME communities about mental health issues.

Better care and treatment

Fundamental to Everybody's Business is this message: that the mental health needs of older people are the business of everyone working in health and social care services who has contact with older people. The reality of risk of mental health problems in this age group is that everyone, from home care and residential care services through to general hospital nursing staff, needs to be alert to the mental well-being of their clients and know how and where to refer them for specialist assessment and treatment, where appropriate. They also need basic grounding in the principles of person-centred care and a recovery-based approach: too often older people are written off as too old to make changes that will improve the quality of their life.

Primary care

Salford Mental Health Services and Salford & Trafford Health Authority have tried to improve service provision for older adults with mild to moderate mental health problems by improving awareness of primary care (GP) staff about the mental health needs of older people. They have introduced:

- accredited training for primary care nurses in identifying and the initial management of mental health problems in older people, including dementia and depression

- pilot NVQ-accredited training schemes for social workers and home carers

- protocols to help primary care staff make appropriate referrals

- improved access to psychology, occupational therapy and counselling

- mental health/primary care liaison to promote mental health in older people and improve liaison between primary care and specialist mental health care services.

This is particularly important for staff working in community settings, including residential care home staff and staff working in GP practices. There is plentiful evidence of the failure by GPs and residential care homes to be alert to older people's mental well-being. Too often attention is focused on people's functional needs, such as feeding, washing, dressing and mobility (Stewart *et al*, 2003). But if older people in residential care are asked what is important to them, what makes for 'quality of life', it's how they feel mentally (Hoe *et al*, 2006).

Residential care home support

In South Gloucestershire a specialist service offers support and advice to residential home care staff. The service comprises a full-time mental health nurse and part-time approved social worker (with specialist training in mental health), supported by a consultant old-age psychiatrist. The team links with ten homes in the area and can be requested by care homes to work with residents who may be at risk of admission to hospital or transfer to another home because of deteriorating mental health and behavioural difficulties. They can also help when a resident is being discharged from hospital back to the care home. The nurse helps care staff assess the individual and advises on their care. The social worker provides training, support and advice to the whole staff team on ways to make the environment more suitable, through assistive technology (door alarms, etc) and signage, décor and fittings.

For staff working in residential care, this means having and taking the time to organise activities, find out what the individuals in their care enjoy, introduce them to new activities within their capabilities, and ensure they stay in touch with friends and family and make new friends within the home. This is, fundamentally, about good person-centred care, which should guide all health and social care practice.

Supporting home care workers

In Bristol the older people's mental health service has introduced training for its home care workers so they are better equipped and more confident in working with older people with mental health needs living independently in the community. Training is provided on mental health and its impact on people's behaviour, recognising when mental health needs may be changing, and managing challenging behaviours. A community psychiatric nurse attached to the scheme provides the training and on-going one-to-one consultation for the home care workers, and will also visit clients with the home care worker to observe and advise.

The Social Care Institute for Excellence (SCIE) has published an online practice guide on Assessing the Mental Health Needs of Older People (SCIE, 2006). This is based on the principle outlined in the Securing Better Mental Health for Older Adults document: that older people can be helped to recover from mental health problems, and should be offered medication and any other treatments, such as counselling, that would automatically be considered for a younger person. The aim of assessment should always be to promote independence and minimise distress.

However, sadly, at the other end of the scale there is equally pressing evidence of over-treatment: that older people (particularly in residential care homes) are being prescribed powerful sedatives to manage difficult and disruptive behaviours (Burstow 2003; 2005). Prescription of antipsychotics to older people has increased four-fold in recent years (Burstow, 2005). It has been estimated that as many as 25,000 nursing home residents are being sedated when there is no medical need, and being given 'cocktails' of several drugs, despite national guidance requiring annual medication reviews for all older people taking medication (Burstow, 2005). These powerful sedatives can cause severe side effects, restricting older people's independence and mobility so they are made still more dependent, as well as potentially leading to adverse drug reactions, and to falls. Often the problem is lack of staff in residential care homes, and a lack of training among care staff in communicating and working with older people with dementia and challenging behaviours. The priority then becomes containment, exacerbating the distress of the individual.

There is also evidence that older people are subjected more frequently than younger adults to invasive treatments such as ECT (electro-convulsive therapy). Use of ECT to treat depression in older people is double that of all other age groups: in one survey 46% of patients given ECT were aged 65+ (Mind, 2005). Yet there is evidence that ECT can exacerbate confusion and memory loss, and that other side effects associated with the treatment are heightened in older people (Mind, 2005). ECT should only be used in a single, short course to gain fast, short-term improvement of severe symptoms after all other treatment options have failed, or when the situation is thought to be life-threatening – and never as long-term, continuous therapy (NICE, 2003).

Holistic approach

Age Concern Warwickshire has set up a mental health support centre for older people with mild and moderate mental health problems, where they can meet as a group and take part in a range of individual and group therapeutic and social activities. Referrals come from GPs, community mental health teams, social services and GPs. The older people decide what they want to do, supported by volunteers and staff. The service aims to encourage positive mental health and independence and to meet people's psychological, physical, spiritual and emotional needs in one location. It also provides a contact point for information and support for carers.

Capacity and consent

Consent to treatment is an important issue. Older people (unless they are sectioned under the Mental Health Act) must give informed consent to any treatment. The new Mental Capacity Act, which comes into force in 2007, sets out the legal rights of older people who, because of dementia for example, are deemed not mentally capable of making decisions about their care themselves. It is important that staff working in older people's care services know about this new law and what it requires of them.

The Mental Capacity Act 2005

The Mental Capacity Act is based on five key principles:

- every adult has the right to make his or her own decisions and must be assumed to have capacity to do so unless proved otherwise

- whenever possible, people must be supported to make their own decisions

- just because an individual makes what might be seen as an unwise decision, they should not be treated as lacking capacity to make that decision

- anything done or decisions made under the Act for or on behalf of a person who lacks capacity must be done in their best interests

- anything done for or on behalf of a person who lacks capacity should be the least restrictive of their basic rights and freedoms.

It introduces new provisions to enable care staff to make decisions about people's day-to-day care and health needs.

It introduces a new Lasting Power of Attorney, whereby a person can appoint someone to take decisions on their behalf about (for example) major health and medical matters, welfare issues (like housing) and financial matters. It also introduces a system of court-appointed deputies, who can take decisions for a person if they have not been able to appoint their own LPA.

These individuals must always act in the person's best interests, and must always try to act on what the person's wishes would be, from what they know of the person and from asking friends, family and others who know them well.

It also introduces a new right to make advance decisions about any medical treatment the person does not want (even when it might be life-saving), which doctors have to respect.

A new independent mental capacity advocate (IMCA) service will also be created, to help people who have no family or friends make decisions about medical treatment and welfare issues.

(See www.dca.gov.uk/menincap/legis.htm)

Conclusion

In some places there are very good services that are trying to address the problems outlined above. But these are the exception, not the norm. Services for older people with mental health needs are chronically under-resourced, and are likely to remain so while older people are marginalised and devalued in our society. But, as individuals and in the organisations for which they work, health and care workers can make an enormous difference to the quality of life of older people with mental frailty, often by the most simple acts of human kindness and respect.

More examples of good practice in meeting older people's mental health needs can be found on the CSIP/NIMHE website at http://nimhe.org.uk

References

Burstow P (2003) *Keep taking the medicine* 2. London: Liberal Democrats.

Burstow P (2005) *Keep taking the medicine* 3. London: Liberal Democrats.

CSIP (2005) *Everybody's business: integrated mental health services for older adults. A service development guide.* London: Department of health.

Department of Health (2001) *National service framework for older people.* London: Department of Health.

Department of Health (2005) *Securing better mental health for older adults.* London: Department of Health.

Healthcare Commission (2006) *Living well in later life: a review of progress against the national service framework for older people.* London: Healthcare Commission.

Hoe J, Hancock G, Livingston G *et al* (2006) Quality of life of people with dementia in residential care homes. *British Journal of Psychiatry* **188** 460-464.

Joseph Rowntree Foundation (2004) *Black and minority ethnic older people's views on research findings.* York: JRF.

MHF/Age Concern (2006) *Promoting mental health and well-being in later life: a first report from the UK Inquiry into Mental Health and Well-being in Later Life.* London: MHF, 2006.

Mind (2005) *Access all ages.* London: Mind.

NICE (2003) *The clinical effectiveness and cost effectiveness of electroconvulsive therapy (ECT) for depressive illness, schizophrenia, catatonia and mania.* London: NICE.

RCPsych (2006) *Raising the standard: specialist services for older people with mental illness.* London: RCPsych, 2006.

SCIE (2006) *Assessing the mental health needs of older people. Online guide.* London: SCIE. (www.scie.org.uk)

Seabrooke V, Milne A (2004) *Culture and care in dementia: a study of the Asian community in north west Kent.* London: Mental Health Foundation/Alzheimer's and Dementia Support Services.

Singleton N, Aye Maung N, Cowie A *et al* (2002) *Mental health of carers.* London: HMSO.

Social Exclusion Unit (2006) *A sure start to later life: ending inequalities for older people.* London: Office of the Deputy Prime Minister.

Stewart K, Worden A, Challis D (2003) Assessing the needs of older people in care homes. *Nursing and Residential Care* **5** (1) 22-25.

Chapter 8
Closing the therapeutic triangle: carer support and why it isn't happening

Alan Worthington

Imagine the board of a supermarket chain that praised the management for the quality of its customer surveys, while the goods on offer were of poor quality and past their sell-by date. Six years after its launch, standard 6 of the national service framework for mental health (Department of Health, 1999) has not been successful in stimulating imaginative solutions for carers. Performance targets are based on carer assessments when they should be rewarding the creation of services that promote greater carer awareness, engagement and support.

Carer networks welcomed the arrival of the national service framework, and particularly standard 6, which expanded the brief of the Carers Services and Recognition Act (CASRA), 1995. Many professionals had rejected the latter on the grounds that it created hurdles for the carer to negotiate and it was unethical to offer people assessments when there were inadequate resources to meet their needs. CASRA required the carer's needs to be assessed only if a care manager was carrying out an assessment of their relative and if it was considered that they (the carer) were providing a 'significant amount' of care. In mental health, 'significant' proved difficult to define. Resources to fund the commissioning of services were limited. As a consequence, some carers summed up this flawed legislation as 'few services and very little recognition'.

The arrival of NSF standard 6 appeared to address some of these difficulties and the rationale showed understanding about caring:

> 'All individuals who provide regular and substantial care for a person on CPA should:
> ▪ have an assessment of their caring, physical and mental health needs, repeated at least on an annual basis
> ▪ have their own written care plan, which is given to them and implemented in discussion with them.' (Department of Health, 1999)

The rationale behind this was that carers play a vital role; therefore providing help, advice and services to carers is one of the best ways of helping people with mental health problems. It acknowledged the strain and responsibilities placed upon the carer and their impact on the carer's health. It directed that carer's needs be assessed and that they receive easy to read information about the help available and the services provided, including medication, other treatment and care, and what to do and who to contact in a crisis. A written care plan would be agreed with the carer and reviewed annually, and 'performance would be monitored by improved satisfaction and confidence among carers about local services'. The lead responsibilities were to lie with social services departments, working in partnership with health and other agencies.

There emerged at once a flaw with standard 6. A strategy that depends on an assessment that in turn relies on a user being on CPA (the Care Programme Approach) assumes that there is consistency about the process whereby people enter the mental health service, become users and are offered care management. Many people do not reach the CPA threshold yet still receive substantial care from family and friends who are carers. Many arrive slowly at the point of being assessed and treated but prior to this point have carers with considerable needs. In the same way that CASRA made carers jump through hoops, NSF standard 6, if applied rigorously, excludes some carers.

There are two further very major issues arising from standard 6, neither of them yet resolved. The first is the vexed issue of confidentiality; the second is the carer assessment itself.

Confidentiality

Important issues lie behind the statement in standard 6 concerning 'the sharing of information', which includes the following caveat (in very small print): 'The service user's consent should always be explicitly sought before information is passed to their carer.'

This endorses the professionals' codes of conduct about client confidentiality. There can be little disagreement with this principle, but the term is vague and general. Does this refer to all information? This approach would automatically prevent a large number of carers having access to the information, knowledge and support they needed to be able to care for their relative. It would also fail to promote good communication between clinician and carer.

The caveat continues: 'If the service user is incapacitated, information may be passed to the carer if it is in the service user's best interests.' Again there is a lack of clarity. What does 'incapacitated' mean? An inpatient admission can be an extremely challenging time for user and carer. The capacity of the user may be poor but not absent. At this time the carer's need for support and explanations is extremely high. These caveats remain as a challenge to carers and professionals. Can confidences be held on all sides and effective communication still take place?

Since the arrival of standard 6 care for people with mental health problems has increasingly moved to community services. The total burden on informal carers has increased. Many of the challenges and rewards of home-based care are hidden behind closed doors. In some families support takes hours each day; in others short inputs create a stimulus towards recovery or staying well. It is extremely difficult to quantify objectively the importance of what carers contribute. Can CPA be detached from the process of providing carer support? Can the pitfalls of trying to define 'regular or substantial care' be avoided by offering support to all carers of people with mental health problems?

Carers are likely to know the person when s/he is well, and so can recognise quite subtle early changes. Clinicians need to be willing to receive this information, in order that interventions can be made and disruption to lives avoided.

In the therapeutic triangle of professional, user and carer there appears to be an illogical imbalance in observing confidences. There is great emphasis on the professionals' codes of conduct with regard to service users, but carers are entitled to respect for their confidences too; these should not be passed to the service user. Records and letters from carers should not be kept in patients' files; they should be stored separately. Unfortunately there are instances when sensitive information is released that can damage relationships within the family and may lead to risk of physical harm.

To be effective in carrying out their roles and responsibilities, carers need information and advice. For example, they are unlikely to be able to distinguish between the symptoms of illness and medication side effects. Information of a general type lies outside the bounds of confidentiality and should be available. Carers also need advice on how to deal with very unusual situations that lie outside normal experience.

It is a matter of great regret that, although standard 6 was intended to be supportive of carers, it has totally failed to tease out the confidentiality issue, and this has continued to give staff anxieties when sharing information with carers. Too many have opted for the safe solution, using confidentiality as a device to block engagement.

In response to this void, professionals in partnership with carer networks have created guidelines for sharing information. For example the Royal College of Psychiatrists' Partners in Care campaign (see www.rcpsych.ac.uk/campaigns/partnersincare.aspx) has produced three checklists – for professionals, carers and users – setting out the questions the professional should ask the carer, and the carer and user might wish to ask the professional. This reinforces the concept of a therapeutic triangle in which the carer receives knowledge and strategies, and good communication is encouraged between all three. Another publication, from the National Co-ordinating Centre for NHS Service Delivery and Organisation (SDO), sets out the key principles that should guide the development of local information sharing policies, based on research into users', carers' and professionals' views (SDO, 2006). Such policies, say the researchers who produced this briefing, are all too often absent but could make a great contribution by clarifying what each side can expect and is able to offer.

Carer assessments

Delivery of standard 6 has been dominated by assessment. There is major inconsistency in the design and delivery of this process across England, with each social services department creating its own solution. A good carer's assessment benefits from a worker being wholly sympathetic to the carer's situation. It can be difficult for those workers who are normally and closely involved with service users to switch to take on the carer's perspective in an assessment.

Workers doing assessments must be experienced because carers can easily deflect the assessment process to looking at the user's needs, losing sight of their own needs. Workers need to be familiar with the challenges and dilemmas that the carer may be facing, and probe beyond the obvious issues.

Managers, too, may have their blind spots, particularly in assuming that receiving an assessment will be high on the carer's agenda. For example, what of the carer who says: 'Thanks for the offer but I'm worn out. I'm desperate for a break but can't face going through the whole story again'?

When an assessment has been done, what happens to the assessment paperwork? The assessment may identify issues that are in the domain of the NHS, but the carer support worker holding the assessment information may not be an NHS employee. Some do not have a clear route for reporting unmet needs. Only recently have joint health and social care appointments been made to these posts. Better links are needed to bring together information from different sources about carers and deliver it to service commissioners.

In service discussions, there is great emphasis on evidence-based services. Carers identify very similar problems and needs. Any further research into 'what carers need' would be a huge waste of time and money: there are shelves and filing cabinets filled with such research evidence, and still carers get very little in the way of resources.

The following quotes from carer support workers (CSWs) highlight some of the obstacles to improving carer support and illustrate the tendency of services to create boundaries between the different agencies.

> 'In our service, all carers must enter through the assessment gate before we can work with them.'

> 'In many localities doing assessments is simply a number crunching exercise.'

'Letters were sent out offering assessments to all the known carers. For many, this was unnecessary and inappropriate so they declined. There is now a new performance target: "Assessment offered and declined".'

'We can only carry out a carer's assessment if the service user is a client of the trust.'

'I couldn't help the carer because she lives in my patch but the service user lives in the next county.'

'I keep the carers assessment paperwork in my desk drawer. My line manager and her boss don't want to see it.'

'It gives us a big problem if the service user refuses a care plan meeting because we can't treat the carer as a client.'

Perhaps the most worrying aspect of the assessment process is a systemic failure to address the unmet needs of carers, and to record, collate and use these needs as the basis for service development and commissioning.

Good practice

A West Country mental health charity has been managing CSWs for 15 years. The service is open to any carers in adult mental health services. Carers can self-refer or be referred by statutory workers; the only proviso is that either the user or carer must live in the area. Carers receive the total range of support services, whether or not they have had an assessment or the user is on CPA.

Positive outcomes

One positive outcome of the arrival of standard 6 was an increase in the number of CSWs. Previously the creation of CSW posts was haphazard – dependent largely on locality managers' budgets and heavy lobbying by carers. At that time, carer support appointments were not considered the remit of the health services. In 2004 the Department of Health provided resources for 700 additional CSWs yet, as Louis Appleby, national director for mental health, has acknowledged (Appleby, 2004), there has been too little progress to report towards the target of supporting carers.

Carers have consistently reported their needs as:

- emotional support
- help in finding appropriate information
- coping strategies and dealing with guilt, stigma and a sense of loss.

In addition, some identify a need for respite breaks and support with work and financial matters.

However, the central issues common to all carers and a challenge to all who work in mental health are:

- how to make professionals more aware of carers and their needs
- how to ensure better engagement of professionals with carers
- better access to information, coping strategies and support.

A major part of carer support work is 'active listening'. It is therefore very important that all professionals should be aware of their local CSW and signpost carers to their services.

Good practice

CSWs should offer several one-to-one sessions with carers, offering time and opportunity for extended conversations. Initially the meetings may involve emotional accounts of the carer's story. Carers often report that this is the first time they have been given 'quality listening'. The focus can then move to the formal assessment process.

CSWs report that it is often possible to see carers working out their own solutions through these conversations. It may be necessary for them to be supported when meeting clinicians and managers, in order for some of these issues to be resolved.

There is merit in the carers assessment, if it is well designed and executed with skill, and if follow-up services are in place so that carers who ask for help can be assessed and directed to appropriate solutions. But what of those carers who remain outside the services? Some remain unaware of the right to an assessment, while others will shun statutory services because they don't want the stigma they attach to involvement.

What can carers and workers learn from assessments as currently carried out? For carers, the process itself – if done properly – can be of benefit in helping them clarify their needs and talk through solutions. They may become aware of external resources but, most importantly, they may find new resources within themselves.

For the CSW, the assessment may improve engagement with the carer. If the information from assessments is collated, managers, commissioners and auditors can identify unmet needs that could result in a better, more comprehensive service for carers.

There are some encouraging signs that the assessment of carers' needs will be given greater prominence in national policy and practice. For example, the Royal College of Psychiatrists' voluntary accreditation for acute inpatient mental health services (AIMS) scheme (RCPsych, 2006) includes as one of its indicators of quality that 'the principal carer is offered an assessment of their own needs'. This work is being aligned with the Healthcare Commission's annual improvement review of acute inpatient services, offering an opportunity to monitor at national level how well services are putting into practice issues of relevance to carers.

But monitoring the meeting of carers' needs can be done quite simply, by starting from a list of core needs as identified by carers. The services offered to meet those needs would then be the subject of local audit, which could include assessments by carers of the quality of the solutions. This would fit with the standard 6 local milestone for 'improved satisfaction and confidence'.

Conclusion

Carers' needs are still not fully recognised in mental health service provision. Carers are vital partners in the care and support of people with mental health problems. By working with and providing support to carers, services are drawing on an important and currently under-acknowledged resource. One thing I do believe to be true: services should be rewarded not for carrying out carer assessments but for the creation of better services for carers, based on the needs identified from the assessments.

References

Appleby L (2004) *The national service framework for mental health – five years on.* London: Department of Health.

Department of Health (1999) *National service framework for mental health: modern standards and service models.* London: Department of Health.
(www.dh.gov.uk/assetRoot/04/07/72/09/04077209.pdf)

Royal College of Psychiatrists (2006) *Accreditation for acute inpatient mental health services (AIMS).* London: Royal College of Psychiatrists.
(www.rcpsych.ac.uk/crtu/centreforqualityimprovement/aims.aspx)

SDO (2006) *Sharing mental health information with carers: pointers to good practice for providers.* London: National Co-ordinating Centre for NHS Service Delivery and Organisation.
(www.sdo.lshtm.ac.uk/pdf/carers_huxley_briefingpaper.pdf)

Chapter 9
Service user involvement in mental health services: what's the point?

David Crepaz-Keay

Over the last 20 years, service user involvement has moved from being a demand from radical survivor groups to a commonplace requirement of mainstream NHS and social care providers, grant funding bodies and service level agreements between the state and private and voluntary sector provider organisations. Almost no one now challenges the notion that service user involvement is a good thing. But, like so many things that become an accepted part of life, there is the risk that we forget the purpose of service user involvement.

This risk is compounded by a certain amount of confusion about what it is (and indeed what it isn't). There is a distinction to be made between consultation and involvement. Consultation is characterised by a tight framework and is usually consultation on a well-developed entity. There are three distinct types of service user involvement. In its most literal – and most often ignored – form, service user involvement describes people's involvement in their own care and treatment. At the next level up, service user involvement describes the mechanism used by organisations that provide mental health services to directly involve people who use their services in the organisation, delivery and monitoring of those services. And last, at the upper-most level, it refers to the involvement of people who are using, or have used, mental health services in mental health policy development and review of services at a national level.

Guiding principles
In an ideal world there should be seamless movement between these categories: each is inextricably linked to, and builds on, the others, and a shared number of principles underpin all three.

■ **Service user involvement should make things better**
Although the process of being involved may have some benefits, there is little point in putting effort and energy into this simply to tick some box in a contract.

■ **Service user involvement should be inclusive, not exclusive**
It's not about an individual on a committee, it's about people's experience of informing decision-making.

■ **Service user involvement must be accessible**

Talk of 'hard to reach' groups often masks under-resourced or ill thought-out approaches. Language is designed to help communication, not prevent it – clear communication is an essential part of any service user involvement strategy.

■ **Everybody involved should be honest about what they want from it**

If the limits of decision-making are clear, no one will feel duped by what happens next. If service users see this as a way of increasing their skills and experience, this benefit may be built in as part of the deal.

Five simple questions

When contemplating any piece of service user involvement, the following five questions provide a useful guide that will, hopefully, ensure everyone gets what they want from it:

1 what's the point (for me, for them)?
2 who should be involved?
3 involved in what?
4 what's up for grabs (what can and cannot be changed)?
5 is it safe?

Why these questions need answers will unfold as they are applied to each type of involvement.

Involving people in their own care

It always strikes me as odd, but this is undoubtedly the poor relation of the service user involvement family. The point of involving the service user at this level is, surely, self-evident. Most aspects of the mental health system could be significantly improved by constructively involving people in their own care. Involving people in their own care is likely to have a number of benefits: typically, improved outcomes, faster recovery, and longer periods of sustained recovery between crises. Evidence from other branches of medicine suggests treatment plans are more likely to be adhered to and more likely to be effective if the person receiving the treatment is involved in the project (Letfey & Wishner, 1999). It seems reasonable to assume mental health care would be the same. If people understand what is wrong with them, what those treating them propose to do about it, how what they propose is intended to work, what the side effects are, what the disbenefits as well as benefits are likely to be, the risks and the alternatives, they are undoubtedly more likely to follow the course. At the most extreme end of service failure, people seeking help and being denied it is a common feature in reports into serious incidents involving people with a psychiatric diagnosis (see, for example, Ritchie *et al*, 1994). One of the key barriers to involvement at this level is the continuing professional delusion that people with a psychiatric diagnosis, by the nature of their diagnosis, lack insight into their condition. There is plentiful evidence that, given the opportunities outlined above, this is very much not the case. Insight too often gets taken to mean acceptance of someone else's conceptualisation of the situation and its remedy.

The answers to the second and third questions should be evident, though the third is clearly constrained by the fourth.

What's up for grabs is one of those crunch points – honesty is the key to getting this right. Offering people choices that simply aren't available is one of the best ways of putting people off getting involved; similarly, asking for people's views and then ignoring them won't encourage them to volunteer their opinions again. In terms of people's own care, it's important to be clear about what is and isn't available, which decisions are fixed and which are dependent on factors outside your and their control.

Safer service user involvement is an underdeveloped field. In the context of individual care, it is important that the risks of not involving people properly are judged alongside more conventional risk issues. People need good information to get involved in a meaningful way. They may need support from others – from peers, family, friends, or advocates. This should not be an adversarial situation; we're talking negotiation here. It has to be pointed out that vast sums of money are spent on training staff in pretty much every aspect of mental health, including service user involvement. Risks associated with involving people in their own care could easily be mitigated by what amounts to education, in the form of proper preparation and ongoing support. In the voluntary sector, the Manic Depression Fellowship has developed proven effective self-management tools and techniques for people with bipolar disorder, but the government's Expert Patient Programme (Department of Health, 2001) – intended to support self-management by people with long-term health conditions – has not been extended in any meaningful way to people with a psychiatric diagnosis.

Involving service users in the services they are using

Involving people in their own care requires (still too often) a seismic shift in the attitudes of mental health professionals and staff. Involving people in the services they use requires an equally seismic structural shift in the organisation, as well as a mind-shift in everyone involved – including the 'involvees'.

Even among service users, the move from wanting more control over how I am treated to how and what services I think should be provided is a leap that most don't make. Why should we? That's why we pay our taxes, so people who are paid to do it, and trained to do it, do it for us. The vast majority of people using mental health services simply want to use them and then get on with their life. But from the point of view of the organisation, service users are a huge, untapped resource: if the organisation is able to provide what users find helpful, in a way they find acceptable, it will unquestionably result in better outcomes for all concerned.

But we are talking here about transforming a system that has been built from top to bottom with the primary aim of delivering what experts decide should be provided to passive recipients, who are assumed not to know what is good for them. (This analysis catches the author in generous mood. Much of the system was actually designed to contain people whom society fears or detests. It is no coincidence that the Victorian asylums were populated by unmarried mothers, social misfits and what contemporary societies considered 'undesirables', that the Mental Health Act is disproportionately used on young black men, and it's worth putting a few quid on the wearing of hoodies turning up in some diagnostic criteria before too long.)

So, what do you (the organisation) want out of involving service users in your services? Honestly? If you have a vision of what you want out of services with added user involvement, then articulate it early in the process. This helps service users decide if there's anything in it for them. Then, when service users have told you what they think about your vision, if they suggest changes, then change it. Are you prepared to do so? Welcome to the world of service user involvement – one of the apparent paradoxes, certainly when you start from a low base, is that the more you involve service users, the more criticism you'll get. This simply demonstrates that it's working: that people care about what you're doing and are not afraid to give their views. It's not working if no one disagrees with you. There is an outside chance that this is because your scheme is perfect in every respect; it is much more likely that people either can't be bothered or aren't motivated because they don't think any good will come of it, or you haven't created the conditions in which it feels possible for them to get involved. Alongside those who have never been involved are those who have been bruised by years of involvement with precious little gain. There is a range of incentives that can be offered to overcome this 'involvement fatigue', including money, but the most effective is likely to be demonstrating that things actually do happen, that services do improve in ways that service users want, as a result.

The question of 'who should be involved?' should be relatively straightforward, although there are decisions to be made about people who have used the service and how recent that service use needs to be to be appropriate and useful. The 'in what?' and 'what's up for grabs?' questions are crucial and need to be made explicit from the start. Different skills will be needed for involvement in staff recruitment and in monitoring and evaluation. People need to know what's fixed (policies, budgets, buildings, staffing levels etc) and what can be changed (access hours, types of referral, types of services, colour of paint...), so that time and effort can be applied where they are useful, and aren't wasted on unchangeables. And, of course, so that service users know that their involvement will make a difference where they want it. No one is going to want to spend hours of their life discussing matters they don't consider relevant to their priorities.

Safety is incredible important for this type of involvement. It is easy to underestimate how nervous people get about criticising services or staff on which they rely. Service providers have a history of denial and defensiveness when faced with negative feedback. People may have experienced problems after being critical of services; in less enlightened times some have had them withdrawn; they will be reluctant to take that risk again. Service user involvement also exposes people to involvement burnout. People who get involved and are naturally good at it tend to be leapt on by everyone doing service user involvement. If not carefully handled, this can cause two serious problems: isolating people from their peers, and overloading people with complicated and demanding work without adequate payment or support. Involving people collectively can help, and although it isn't always appropriate to involve groups, involving people in pairs is generally not too difficult.

Involving people in the broader policy environment

Last, and arguably most complex if only because of its larger scale, there is involvement at the policy-making level. This covers a vast range of activities, from involvement in local service planning and review groups through to involvement in government task forces and committees developing policy at national level. It's also the most complicated and controversial area, but the key questions remain a useful guide to getting it right.

The point of involvement will vary with each initiative but service users are readily drawn to national initiatives for a variety of reasons, not least of which is the opportunity to influence decisions that can make a huge difference to thousands of lives. There is no doubt that even the most senior policy maker or practitioner can be moved by personal contact with the results of their decisions.

The question of 'who should be involved?' is one of the most troubling questions at this broader level. Once upon a time, there were strong, if small, national groups of politicised service users with sizeable active memberships who might have been regarded as representative of the greater service user view (although they often had reservations about being seen in this role). But they have dwindled (arguably more so as more organised, centrally funded representative bodies have developed, such as the Department of Health's NIMHE service user involvement structure), and national organisations have had to look to individuals – sometimes styled 'champions', sometimes 'experts by experience' – to fill this gap. Consequently, great weight (in every sense) can be placed on the personal views of a very small number of people. For some positions of this type, organisations now go through a formal recruitment process, even for unpaid roles. A recruitment process forces the recruiter to think about the role and type of person they're looking for; it gives them an opportunity to create a transparent process; they can even involve service users in the recruitment process. It also, of course, allows them to pick the person who best serves their ends.

There are often calls for some form of democratic process for this type of involvement. This, we know from experience, raises as many problems as those it is intended to solve. Probably the biggest problem is the lack of a natural constituency or electorate. It's simple enough for a constituted charity or company to define its members, but for a government department, public service regulator or commissioning body, there is no such simple answer. One nutter, one vote may sound attractive in principle, but it is hardly practicable.

It's at times like these that service users need to act collectively. Not in the manner of a 1970s trade union with a privileged individual wielding a block vote on behalf of the brothers, but in a way that promotes the voices of those kept most silent. Previous attempts to speak collectively at a national level have achieved a significant amount; particularly in getting survivor training established for professionals and in setting up training the trainers initiatives. But the number of individuals actually involved was quite small, and came from a relatively narrow cross-section of society. Tomorrow's network needs to be much more inclusive – a network of networks from across the country, reaching people wherever they live and helping those without a local group to network in other ways. This is not about 'representativeness' but about reflecting the broad range of experiences of people using (or needing and not getting) services today.

What's up for grabs? There are a number of issues that can only work at a national level, but there are many stakeholders, and anyone planning service user involvement needs to be really clear about what could change. I have been to countless national meetings where almost everything has been decided in advance by a small subset. Sometimes a presence at the table is all you get, and people will need to decide whether that's worth having. Sometimes it's part of a longer game; you just need to check your own motivations and avoid becoming part of a cosy élite.

For those that do get involved at this level, safety is again a vital issue. People can quickly become isolated from their peers and find themselves standing between, on the one side, a whole government department and, on the other, disgruntled (and worse) service users convinced that they've sold their souls for a finger buffet (or a pharma- funded trip to an island paradise...). No one should have to face these pressures alone. Nor should they feel anything but honourable if they admit defeat and return to more comfortable territories. A national network could support a range of individuals and groups, and would help make this level of involvement a safer thing to do.

Conclusion

To shift from the belief that service user involvement is right and proper to making it happen in a meaningful way requires time, organisation, patience and understanding, support and, above all, a budget. Too many service user involvement initiatives have failed because they are not adequately resourced.

Primary care trusts (or commissioners in any future service reconfiguration) will clearly have a role in building capacity here. A recent (2006) initiative from the Department of Health to fund broader patient and public involvement in health though Local Involvement Networks (LINks) is worth watching (Department of Health, 2006). But generally, it seems everybody wants service user involvement but not everyone is so keen to pay for it.

If you want value for money in service user involvement, the formula is simple. Be clear about what you want it to do, don't confuse consultation with involvement, quick and cheap is likely to cost you more in the long run, and nine times out of ten you're better off building a good relationship with a high quality local supplier.

References

Department of Health (2001) *The expert patient: a new approach to chronic disease management for the 21st century.* London: Department of Health. www.expertpatients.nhs.uk

Department of Health (2004) *A stronger local voice: a framework for creating a stronger local voice in the development of health and social care services.* London: Department of Health.

Department of Health (2006) *A stronger local voice: a framework for creating a stronger local voice in the development of health and social care services.* London: Department of Health.

Letfey K, Wishner WJ (1999) Beyond 'compliance' is 'adherence'. *Diabetes Care* **22** (4).

Ritchie J, Dick D, Lingham R (1994) *The report of the inquiry into the care and treatment of Christopher Clunis.* London: HMSO.

Recommended reading

HASCAS (2005) *Making a real difference: strengthening service user and carer involvement in NIMHE.* London: HASCAS. (http://kc.nimhe.org)

Together (2006) *Service users together: a guide for involvement.* Brighton: Pavilion. (www.pavpub.com)

Wallcraft J (2003) *On our own terms.* London: Sainsbury Centre for Mental Health. (www.scmh.org.uk)

Chapter 10
What are we waiting for? choice in the mental health system

Liz Main

'Patient choice' is suppose to define the modern NHS. The government says it is putting personal choice at the heart of its health service reform agenda, and creating a 'patient-led NHS' (Department of Health, 2005). In reality, for those of us who use mental health services, choice remains limited to what the system chooses to offer us, not what we as individuals consider we need and want.

The patriarchal nature of the mental health system has previously made it near impossible for people who use mental health services to exercise choice in the way most people understand the meaning of the word. Not only do we lack choice over the type of treatment we receive, where and when we are treated, and the professional who treats us; when we are at our most vulnerable we can be deprived of even the most basic of choices, such as when we can eat or sleep (Prior, 2003).

Where physical health services are beginning to understand that patients are consumers who have the right to information to enable them to make decisions about their health care preferences, mental health service providers rarely interpret 'choice' as relating to personal care. Patients may be involved in drawing up their care packages, but only to the extent that they are asked to agree to what's already been decided; all too frequently people who are less articulate or in a crisis are seen as unable to make realistic choices. Overall, the mental health system lacks the capacity and flexibility to provide an individualised service that can give users a real role in shaping the support that will enable their recovery (Rankin, 2005). In an over-burdened system, there is little capacity to allow patients to choose where they want to be treated in a crisis, for example, or who they want to treat them (and most don't know they have the right to do this). The 'choose and book' system allowing people to schedule a convenient appointment is only just being introduced to mental health. So even the most basic mechanisms for enabling patient choice are not in place for mental health service users.

There are no nationally monitored waiting lists in the mental health system, but that doesn't mean you can get a bed in a psychiatric hospital (or, better still, in a crisis house) when you think you need one, or that you won't have to wait months to see a psychotherapist. It's just that the Department of Health doesn't set targets for mental health trusts as it does for the general health and primary care sectors, so the unmet need for treatment remains hidden.

Bringing about choice in mental health doesn't just rely on these practicalities, however. A radical change in attitude and culture is needed: one that recognises the right of service users to take control of their own care, and helps them do so. Too often choice in mental health care is seen as giving users a choice of what colour to paint the walls of a building, rather than what happens in that building.

When I first came into contact with NHS mental health services I was outraged by the dehumanisation I and other patients were expected to endure. One of my first experiences was of being called out of a bath to see a junior doctor immediately, with no prior notice that he wished to see me. I didn't even know I might be seen, let alone when and by whom. Yet when I asked to see him in the following days and weeks, I would usually be fobbed off and told he was too busy. It became clear that when and how I was treated was his choice, not mine.

It was the consultant's choice too, to change my medication without telling me. Lining up for medication one day I was given not my usual white tablet but a coloured capsule. When I queried this, my chart was checked and I was informed this was my new medication. No mention of what it was or why it had been prescribed, or of the side effects it later had. Just an expectation that I would swallow it down.

When I was discharged, I was told where I would see my consultant, although I later found out I could have seen him at a variety of venues. Appointments were sent to me without consultation on times. The assumption was made that I was available.

Seven years on, some things have improved, but too often that is down to enlightened individual practitioners, rather than evidence of genuine change in attitudes and practices. The assumption remains that people with mental health problems either can't or don't want to make decisions. Choice is there for those who know their rights and are prepared to exercise them, but the more vulnerable people are left with no information on what they can choose and how. And for those whose experience of mental illness and its treatment has left them utterly disempowered and without confidence, there is no help with making decisions if they are ever allowed to do so.

What do we want?

Perhaps this is not surprising, given that in setting out the NHS choice agenda the government has more or less ignored mental health. In 2003 it launched a consultation on choice, responsiveness and equity in health care. As part of this consultation it commissioned a mental health expert task group to look specifically at what mental health services users wanted, of which I was a member. We presented the Department of Health with a list of recommendations: a mix of practical measures, cultural change and radical ideas (Prior, 2003). These were ignored in the final report (Department of Health, 2003).

The list wasn't complicated, or very demanding. Information, advocacy, and empowerment topped our recommendations. This is because, while the goal of mental health services is to support people in recovering a life that is meaningful and fulfilling to them, too often services undermine people's capacity to make decisions and take control of their own care. Enabling people to take that control requires information, backed up by advocacy, with services that promote recovery and believe that everyone can achieve independence and a life that has meaning for them. We recommended independent provision of information and advocacy services. There is some provision of advocacy now, but we wanted it to be provided to everyone unless they specifically said they didn't want it, rather than having to ask for it as they do now.

We wanted people to have a choice of where they access mental health services, be it in primary care settings or outside the medical arena – in community or faith settings, for example, to overcome the stigma of using mental health services.

We also recommended the use of legally binding advance directives, to enable people to make choices when they are well about how they wish to be treated in a crisis, and that assistance with preparation of these should be routinely integrated into care planning. (It's interesting that research into use of advance directives has found they made no difference to people's outcomes – because the staff didn't recognise them, didn't encourage patients to use them, and didn't take any notice of them when deciding how to treat them (Papageorgiou *et al*, 2004).)

Other recommendations included access to accredited talking therapies – something every patient survey shows people want, but have to wait months, sometimes years, to get. We recommended informed choice of best-fit medications; a range of alternative and complementary therapies; choice of professional – in particular, key worker – and employment support options. Recommendations on social care suggested people should be given more control over where they live, and that all aspects of an individual's life be considered in care planning.

Our recommendations didn't just come from us. They were in line with what people who use mental health services have been demanding for many years. Research repeatedly shows that people with mental health problems want services that aid recovery and are shaped around their own lives, rather than their activities and aspirations being subsumed by the mental health system. They want services that take account of their gender, culture and ethnicity; they want access to self-management programmes that are orientated towards recovery. The top priorities are a choice of treatments, particularly talking therapies; a say over who they are treated by; and flexibility about and where and when they are treated – but mostly they want quite simply to be listened to and respected (Warner *et al*, 2006).

Choice checklist

Subsequent to the choice consultation, NIMHE published a national framework for choice in mental health services. Our Choices in Mental Health (CSIP, 2005a) sets out the ways in which the mental health system can promote user choice. On paper, the framework and accompanying checklist (CSIP, 2005b) concur with the recommendations of our task group and what individuals say they want: access to talking therapies, alternatives to chemical-based treatments, integration of choice into people's care plans, and information and advocacy to help people get what they have chosen. Yet the reality is that people who use services are yet to benefit (Warner *et al*, 2006).

NIMHE acknowledges that enabling real choice will require massive cultural change, and highlights pockets of good practice (CSIP, 2005b), but this is just a checklist: there's no obligation on services to make any of this available. For example, NIMHE endorses talking therapies, and says that prescriptions should extend beyond medication to include alternatives such as yoga, exercise, aromatherapy, relaxation, nutrition and various other holistic therapies. Dream on.

That said, NIMHE's checklist stops short of offering the breadth of choice that will really meet our needs. When it says talking therapies should be available through either the NHS or the independent/voluntary sector, it doesn't acknowledge the current limitations on availability (Layard, 2005). Increasingly, 'talking therapy' is interpreted as short-term counselling or cognitive behavioural therapy, or even self-help CBT computer programmes. Many people want longer-term psychotherapy to explore issues in their lives underlying their distress. Some groups, particularly black and ethnic minority people, are unlikely to be referred to any talking treatment at all. People who have experienced abuse or trauma may want tailored, specialist psychotherapy. Offering talking therapy is a start, but real choice means providing a range of therapies so people can choose the one that works best for them.

Medication is often used as the first-line or only treatment option for people with mental health problems, even when it is not their preference. However, patients often get little, if any, information on the drugs they are prescribed, and most feel they have no option but to take the pills (Olofinjana & Taylor, 2005). While there are tensions when a person is compelled to take medication under the Mental Health Act, they can be given the opportunity to discuss their medication options and, where possible, to make an informed decision about which drug they take, based on the information given to them about benefits and side effects, and advance directives can be used (Prior, 2003). Given that individuals often know best from experience what drugs suit them, providing choice makes sense from both the patient's and the professional's perspectives.

Making choice happen

Mental health services already have a key mechanism that should ensure people in secondary care are given options: the Care Programme Approach. If this is working, every service user should have a bespoke care package that reflects their own preferences, including the individual they are most frequently in contact with, the agreed therapy and treatment plans, and preferred medication and dosage (if any). Ideally, this will also include an advance directive. Yet the CPA is still less than fully used (Warner, 2005). The Healthcare Commission's 2005 national mental health inpatient survey (Healthcare Commission, 2005) found that only a half were given or offered a copy of their care plan, while one third did not know who their care co-ordinator was. Mental health service providers are going to need to ensure that care planning actually happens, that users are genuinely involved in drawing it up (rather than just being asked to agree what's been decided for them), and better used to draw out and implement what people want and think will help, with more information provided at every level.

The introduction of individual budgets enabling people to purchase their own social care (Department of Health, 2006) offers a huge opportunity for mental health services to make promises of choice a reality. Direct payments already potentially offer that opportunity, but take-up has been slow: research shows that often the block is the attitude of staff who do not believe people with a mental illness diagnosis are capable of managing their own care (Spandler & Vick, 2004). As patients become consumers, we will increasingly want to tailor care packages to our own needs. Clearly NHS providers will not be able to offer us all the options we want, but using individual budgets we should be able to buy the care we want from the NHS, voluntary sector and independent provider organisations. So if I feel a particular therapy would be helpful, I could go to an accredited external provider to buy it, spending the money that the NHS would have spent on its own services. If I thought it would help to have a support worker to take me shopping, or out to the cinema, I could pay someone to do this. Some people might not want the responsibility, but with help they might see that with responsibility comes choice and the chance to get care and support when, where and in a form that is useful to them.

NIMHE's checklist on choice is encouraging, but desperately limited. NIMHE states that: 'Following an assessment, a clinically appropriate personalised care plan is developed with the service user and their carer, family and/or friends. The aim is to support people to make choices within defined limits of the appropriate type, location and providers of their care package.' This clearly returns the power to the clinician, who will ultimately decide what is 'appropriate'. That is giving with one hand and taking away with both: clearly, paternalism is alive and well in the modern NHS.

If people with mental health problems are to be given real control over their care, professionals need to overcome their reluctance to allow patients to make choices that differ from their own. To do this they will have to accept that people can take responsibility for their own well-being, and support them by providing information that is accessible and understandable. Staff may need to encourage individuals to articulate what they want, and work with independent advocates and carers to make this happen. They will need to familiarise themselves with mechanisms for enabling choices in health and social care. Choice (not control) will need to be put at the heart of the CPA, with ongoing monitoring to ensure this is working.

It all comes back to a change in culture: for people with mental health problems choice should be the expectation not the exception.

References

CSIP (2005a) *Our choices in mental health: checklist*. Leeds: CSIP. (http://kc.nimhe.org.uk/index.cfm?fuseaction=Item.viewResource&intItemID=60398)

CSIP (2005b) *Our choices in mental health: a framework for improving choice for people who use mental health services and their carers*. Leeds: CSIP. (http://kc.nimhe.org.uk/index.cfm?fuseaction=Item.viewResource&intItemID=55870)

Department of Health (2003) *Building on the best: choice, responsiveness and equity in the NHS*. London: Department of Health.

Department of Health (2005) *Creating a patient-led NHS: delivering the NHS improvement plan*. London: Department of Health.

Department of Health (2006) *Our health, our care, our say*. London: Department of Health.

Healthcare Commission (2005) *Count me in: results of a national census of inpatients in mental health hospitals and facilities in England and Wales*. London: Healthcare Commission.

Layard R (2005) *Therapy for all on the NHS*. Unpublished lecture. London: Sainsbury Centre for Mental Health. (www.scmh.org.uk)

Olofinjana B and Taylor D (2005) Antipsychotic drugs – information and choices: a patient survey. *Psychiatric Bulletin* **29**: 369-371

Papageorgiou A, Janmohamed A, King M *et al* (2004) Advance directives for patients compulsorily admitted to hospital with serious mental disorders: directive content and feedback from patients and professionals. *Journal of Mental Health* **13** (4) 379-388.

Prior C (2003) *Choice, responsiveness and equity. Department of Health mental health task group report*. London: Department of Health. (www.rethink.org/how_we_can_help/campaigning_for_change/rethink_policy_documents/choice.html)

Rankin J (2005) *Mental health in the mainstream: a good choice for mental health*. London: ippr.

Spandler H, Vick N (2004) *Implementing direct payments in mental health: an evaluation*. London: HASCAS.

Warner L (2005) *Back on track? CPA care planning for service users who are repeatedly detained under the Mental Health Act*. London: Sainsbury Centre for Mental Health.

Warner L, Mariathasan J, Lawton-Smith S *et al* (2006) *A review of the literature and consultation on choice and decision-making for users and carers of mental health and social care services*. London: Sainsbury Centre for Mental Health/King's Fund.

Chapter 11
Direct payments and individual budgets: keys to independence

Tina Coldham

Direct payments are cash payments given by local authorities to people eligible for social care (including mental health) services so that they can make their own care arrangements.

The Department of Health defines the purpose of direct payments thus:

> '... to give recipients control over their own life by providing an alternative to social care services provided by a local council. A financial payment gives the person flexibility to look beyond "off the peg" service solutions for certain housing, employment, education and leisure activities as well as for personal assistance to meet their assessed needs. This will help increase opportunities for independence, social inclusion and enhanced self-esteem.' (Department of Health, 2003)

Their aim is:

> '... to give more flexibility in how services are provided to many individuals who are assessed eligible for social services support. By giving individuals money in lieu of social care services people have greater choice and control over their lives, and are able to make their own decisions about how their care is delivered.' (Department of Health: www.dh.gov.uk)

Note the emphasis on independence, social inclusion, self-esteem and choice and control.

Direct payments first came into being in 1997 when the government passed legislation that allowed local authorities to make them available to adults with disabilities.[1] Eligibility was extended to older people in 2000, and to carers of children with disabilities and young people with disabilities aged 16-17 in 2001.[2] Subsequently, in 2003, the government made it a legal duty for local authorities to make direct payments available to eligible users who wanted them.[3]

---

[1] Community Care (Direct Payments) Act 1996
[2] Health and Social Care Act 2001, Section 57(1)
[3] Community Care, Services for Carers and Children's Services (Direct Payments) (England) Regulations 2003

Direct payments can only be used to pay for social care services. They cannot be used to buy in personal health care – although the line between health and social care services is notoriously unclear where mental health is concerned. People with mental health problems have always been eligible for direct payments – other than some people subject to certain sections of the Mental Health Act 1983 (Department of Health, 2003).

However the numbers of mental health service users using direct payments to pay for their social care needs has been famously low. In 2005 only three quarters of local authorities in England were providing direct payments to people with mental health needs, and only five authorities reported more than 20 mental health service users of direct payments (Department of Health, 2006). The most recent figures show that of 33,760 people receiving direct payments, just 1,136 were people with mental health problems. The largest group of DP users are people with physical disabilities (nearly 12,500), followed by older people (7,566) (CSCI, 2006).

The reasons for this low take-up are many – but there is general agreement (Newbigging & Lowe, 2005; CSCI, 2006) that a major block is the failure by local authorities and social care staff to encourage take-up. A recent Commission for Social Care Inspection (CSCI) report, for example, highlights '… inconsistencies in local procedures… confusing terminology, unnecessary paperwork, bureaucracy and unreasonable criteria' (CSCI, 2006). The report also criticises the lack of information and staff support to help people use direct payments: often people are deterred because they don't feel able to take on the responsibility for employing a personal assistant, and social services staff don't know enough about direct payments to help them.

Denise Platt, chair of the Commission for Social Care Inspection, wrote this in the foreword to a CSCI report on direct payments:

> '… the problems surrounding the implementation of direct payments are, in part, simply a failure of imagination. A genuinely progressive initiative is under way, signalling a programme of change for the whole of social care. We all need to work together to make the changes happen.' (CSCI, 2006)

Why direct payments?

Frances Hasler, a prominent disability and direct payments campaigner, has said this about direct payments, and to me it says it all:

> 'Direct payments are a means to an end and that end is independent living.' (cited in Glasby & Littlechild, 2002)

Independent living is a concept that was born in 1973 when three severely disabled people enrolled to attend university in Berkeley, California. All were wheelchair users and they were supported by personal assistants (PAs). After university they wanted to be able to use their education to get jobs and live ordinary lives, instead of being consigned to a care home. So they then went on to form the first Centre for Independent Living (CIL), which was owned and run by and for disabled people. From these small beginnings grew a whole new disability rights movement that has since spread across the world.

In the UK, the independent living movement also emerged from a group of physically disabled people who were living in a Hampshire care home and were fed up with the prospect of being institutionalised for life. They wanted to be part of the wider community to which they felt they belonged and to which they wanted to contribute. Their fight for freedom from institutionalisation in the early 80s changed the way people with disabilities were regarded by society. The concept that society disables people with disabilities by not making it possible for them to live ordinary lives and by discrimination and social exclusion has now become commonplace.

To me, independent living is about being a part of the community and about reaching your potential as an individual. I believed this before I had mental health problems, and I still do now, when I am living with those mental health problems. This is a philosophy dearly held by people throughout the disability movement, and is based on four key assumptions:

■ all human life is of value

■ anyone, whatever their impairment, is capable of exercising choices

■ people who are disabled by society's reaction to physical, intellectual and sensory impairment and to emotional distress have the right to assert control over their lives

■ disabled people have the right to participate fully in society. (Morris, 1993)

This applies to people with mental health problems just as much as it does to those with physical and intellectual disabilities. For people with mental health problems, I would translate this as:

■ we want to be valued for who we are, however weird and wonderful that might seem at times

■ we can exercise choice, and we know what we want in our lives, given the right help

■ the real problem users and survivors face is stigma and discrimination; this limits our acceptance in wider society and makes it harder for us to be a part of it and take control over our own lives

■ we have the right to be active members of society and not be locked away, out of sight, out of mind, anymore.

To me, independent living holds the key to how direct payments can help to liberate users and survivors from the mental health system and the turmoil of their ill health, and help them live their own lives, in the ways they want and with the support they say they need, rather than being passive recipients of what other people think they should have and be allowed to do.

Obtaining direct payments

There is no definitive list of what you can and cannot buy with your direct payment. That is important: a definitive list – which by its nature would tend to be prescriptive – would inevitably eat away the very core of the user's choice and control. So long as the user defines the independent living 'end' they have in mind for themselves, direct payments holds out the possibility that they can purchase what they believe they need to get to that 'end'.

We know, from an evaluation of a national pilot to implement direct payments in mental health, that users and survivors use direct payments in many different ways: for social support, domestic support, transport, leisure, personal care, education, arts, respite, child minding, therapeutic activities of all kinds, and night sits (Spandler & Vick, 2004). They can be particularly useful for people from black and minority ethnic groups, who can hire personal assistants from their own cultures and backgrounds who speak their language and understand their cultural needs (Newbigging & Lowe, 2005). Statutory services have been notoriously bad at making special provision for people from minority ethnic groups.

This is what one Asian carer said about the way direct payments had transformed her son's life:

> 'We have been asking for over two years for an Asian social worker and social services haven't helped us. We just want Asian people who can give a service to him… We didn't have anyone coming round, no visitors… The personal assistant just comes and talks to him and tries to go out with him. It takes so long just starting to say "Hello".'
> (Newbigging & Lowe, 2005)

Generally people use direct payments to pay for someone to provide help with daily living, like a personal assistant (PA) to help with managing their home, or going shopping, or going out with them to the cinema or other social and leisure activities, for example. They do this either directly as an employer or through an agency.

Some local authorities have a designated officer or team of people appointed specifically to support uptake of direct payments. In other places this role is taken by a Centre for Independent Living (CIL). Direct payments workers assist users to understand their options and the system, and help with assessments and putting individual direct payments packages together. In my experience it's best when a CIL worker is involved, as they can give care co-ordinators a firm steer in understanding what direct payments are all about. This is often invaluable to users as direct payments challenges so many of the entrenched notions mental health workers can have about people's capacity and capability to manage their own care.

My meanderings around the system as a user, and experience working from that perspective, have led me to the conclusion that 'risk' is a dirty and profoundly negative word in mental health. So many practitioners simply will not take 'positive' risks with users because they are afraid of things going wrong, and then being blamed and lambasted in the press. Users have every right to ask: how on earth can practitioners help me to be positive about life and conquer my own fears and torments if they are operating from such a negative stance? To pose another question: if I am well enough to live outside hospital under no Mental Health Act section, what gives services the right to dictate how I live? All things being equal, surely I – as the person using the service – should have the final word on what will help me most – and direct payments should be a pathway to my liberation!

At a systems level, the national service framework for mental health (which sets out the government targets for mental health service improvement) does not mention direct payments (Department of Health, 1999). This is unfortunate because the progress of service delivery is for the most part measured against this 10-year plan. I have had a care co-ordinator say to me, 'If it's not in the NSF why should I bother?' Local authorities have now been made accountable for making direct payments available to more people, and their progress is measured, which has given some impetus for implementation. However, anecdotally, we know that in practice both the law and government guidance encouraging direct payment use in mental health is regularly flouted. I find it obscene that services and practitioners can get away with this. This is why the message of independent living cannot be shouted loudly enough.

The advantage of direct payments is that the recipient is in control and can choose to have what they want, and when. Choice and control are the watchword in implementing direct payments just as they are now in government health and social care policies. You are not reliant on limited and sometimes stigmatising day services. You don't have to wait until they can fit you into their schedules. Direct payments can help to set users and survivors free. Free from revolving door hospital admissions, free from statutory services, free to integrate more fully into society. Direct payments have, literally, liberated some of our physically disabled colleagues from dire residential care homes.

Individual budgets
Under the social care white paper Our Health, Our Care, Our Say (Department of Health, 2006b), the government has made clear it wants to see many more people

take up direct payments, and this has now been made a measure of local authorities' performance, under the CSCI national star rating checks. It also announced the roll out of an expanded version of direct payments, known as individual budgets.

The principles of independent living, of 'choice and control', are also at the heart of individual budgets (IB). In fact, this way of planning support is especially enabling to the user as it puts them at the centre of the whole care planning process. It allows people to express their needs 'up front' and implicitly recognises that they are best placed to understand how those needs can and should be met.

Individual budgets differ from direct payments in that they allow for monies from other sources of government funding to be included in the pot. They include local authority social services, disability equipment, Access to Work and independent living funds, disabled facilities grants and the Supporting People housing support programme. This joining up of money can facilitate a much more joined up package that can meet many more kinds of care and support needs.

The plan is that people eligible for an individual budget will be told how much money in total they can have each year to pay for all their social care needs, as covered by the funds listed above. This will be held on their behalf rather like a bank account, and they can either use it like a direct payment, or take the services offered by their local authority (or other provider body), or a mix of both (Department of Health, 2006b). They can also nominate someone to help them with their individual budget: a broker or advocate, family or friends.

The ethos of this is that it helps movement towards a partnership model of working between the user, the people around them and statutory care services. It also takes some of the responsibility away from having to employ your own personal assistant, if people are frightened by this.

Individual budgets have been piloted in some local authorities for some people with disabilities (including a few people with mental health problems) as 'self-directed support', under a government scheme known as In Control.[4] Response to an evaluation of the very first pilot schemes (In Control, 2005) were very positive. People said they were very happy with the control they had over their lives since they received their individual budget; they, or a family member were now much more likely to be making decisions about their lives, and they were much happier about their care and support, their lives, their homes, and life in the community generally.

In Control provides a template for how individual budgets are going to work. The conventional way that a care package is put together is that a social worker assesses your needs, and draws up a care plan – hopefully involving you, but often this doesn't happen. The care plan says what services you can have – but often these are dictated not by your needs but by what is available and what the local authority thinks it can

---

[4] See www.in-control.org.uk

afford to provide. You then agree and sign the care plan, and your care co-ordinator arranges for this care to be delivered. In practice you have little or no meaningful influence over or involvement in this process. This can be very disempowering.

With individual budgets, a very different model comes into play in which the service user takes more control of the process from the outset.

1 Assessment

The care co-ordinator initiates the process, but the user carries out a self-assessment of their own needs.

2 Plan support

The user develops their own support plan.

3 Agree the plan

The plan is then reviewed by the care co-ordinator and the budget is agreed.

4 Manage individual budget

The money is transferred to the user, or to a nominated agent, or a trust fund, or the local authority manages the budget.

5 Organise support

Support can come from friends/family, personal assistants or from provider organisations.

6 Live life

The user uses the money to provide the support they find most helpful.

7 Review and learn

Review the support and finances with the care co-ordinator and adjust it if there are any changes in needs.

Throughout the whole process, the user is encouraged to take control. Although the care co-ordinator needs to be there for some key decisions, it remains self-directed support. Users can bring in other people to help with assessment and planning and the organisation and delivery of support. This could be family and friends, but also advocates, support brokers, disabled peoples' organisations, and of course the care co-ordinator. But the user leads the process with as much help as they want.

So, the mechanisms are there to give people with disabilities, including mental health problems, a real say in managing their own care needs. The concept and the process present a real challenge to mental health professionals in how they view 'their clients', and to their power base. But this is a real opportunity for people with mental health problems to become active agents in their own lives. Keep the faith and watch this space!

References

Commission for Social Care Inspection (2006) *Direct payments: what are the barriers?* London: CSCI.

Department of Health (1999) *National service framework for mental health: modern standards and service models.* London: Department of Health.

Department of Health (2003) *Direct payments guidance: community care, services for carers and children's services (direct payments) guidance England 2003.* London: Department of Health.

Department of Health (2006a) *Direct payments for people with mental health problems: a guide to action.* London: Department of Health.

Department of Health (2006b) *Our health, our care, our say: a new direction for community services.* London: Department of Health.

Glasby J, Littlechild R (2002) *Social work and direct payments.* Bristol: Policy Press.

In Control (2005) *Qualitative evaluation finding from phase one piloting of In Control: spring 2004 to summer 2005.* (www.in-control.org.uk/downloads/0101_Evaluation_data.ppt)

Morris J (1993) *Independent lives: community care and disabled people.* Basingstoke: Macmillan.

Newbigging K, Lowe J (2005) *Direct payments and mental health: new directions.* York: Joseph Rowntree Foundation.

Spandler H, Vick N (2004) *Direct payments, independent living and mental health – an evaluation.* London: HASCAS.

Chapter 12
New approaches to treating common mental disorders in primary care

Janine Fletcher and Sarah Kendal

Common mental health problems such as depression and anxiety are highly prevalent in primary care: depression, for example, affects up to 2.3 million people (five per cent of the population) at any one time (BMA, 2003). Such mental health problems are estimated to be present in one in four of all GP consultations in the UK (Goldberg & Huxley, 1992).

While these common mental health problems are often considered to be time-limited illnesses, the World Health Organisation (WHO) study of mental disorders found that 33% of people with depression still met the criteria for a depressive diagnosis one year after first seeking treatment (Simon *et al*, 2002). Common mental health problems are also characterised by high rates of relapse and re-occurrence: at least 50% of first episodes of depression are followed by another episode or more, with the risk of further relapse increasing to 70% after the second episode and as high as 90% after a third (Kupfer, 1991).

The impact of common mental health problems on social functioning, physical health and mortality is substantial. They are also a major contributor to global disease burden and disability. In 1990 depression was the fourth most common cause of loss of disability-adjusted life years in the world, and it is projected to become the second most common cause by 2020 (Murray & Lopez, 1996). Anxiety and depression have an adverse impact on employment and are often associated with high rates of absenteeism from work and unemployment. This can create a vicious cycle whereby consequent loss of income and dependence on the welfare state may in turn lead to low self-esteem and difficulties in close personal relationships – themselves factors in depression. Depression is also a contributory factor in two-thirds of all suicides (Sartorius, 2001).

To further complicate matters, people experiencing severe pain from a long-term physical condition may present with depression and anxiety.

The effective management and treatment of common mental health problems is therefore an important issue, especially in primary care where it is estimated that 90-95% of people with depression and anxiety are treated (Department of Health, 2000). However treatment in primary care is often restricted to the prescribing of antidepressants; GPs may feel these are the only intervention available to offer patients. The effectiveness of antidepressant medication has been demonstrated in high quality clinical trials. However treatment is often ineffective as the drugs are frequently not prescribed in sufficiently high doses to be therapeutically effective, or patients do not take the medication as prescribed. This may be for a number of reasons: misinformed beliefs that antidepressants are addictive; a fear of side effects; lack of knowledge that the medication needs to be taken regularly, and simple forgetfulness.

Patients (for these same reasons) often want alternatives to medication: in particular, talking therapies. However access to psychological and/or talking treatments is limited: waiting times of 12 months and longer are reported (Lovell & Richards, 2000).

Government policy

In recent years government policy has addressed some of the issues by focusing attention on improving access to and quality of treatments for patients with common mental health problems.

In 1999 Standard 2 of the national service framework (NSF) for mental health (Department of Health, 1999) set standards for treatment of mental health problems in primary care. It states that any patient who contacts their primary health care team with a common mental health problem should:

- have their mental health needs identified and assessed
- be offered effective treatments.

A practical guide to implementing standard 2 (Gask *et al*, 2003) recommended that primary care trusts:

- organise training for staff
- develop clinical guidelines or prescribing protocols
- provide information to practices about available community resources
- ensure equitable availability of services
- develop partnerships with specialist mental health services
- monitor the quality of services
- make links with social care
- create posts for GPs with a special interest in mental health.

With limited resources and financial support, the primary care sector has struggled to implement these standards and recommendations.

Two key resources have also been provided by NICE, the National Institute for Health and Clinical Excellence: one for depression and one for anxiety (NICE, 2004a; 2004b). Both these guideline documents recommend a 'stepped care model' of service delivery (see *Figure 1*).

Figure 1: The stepped care model for depression

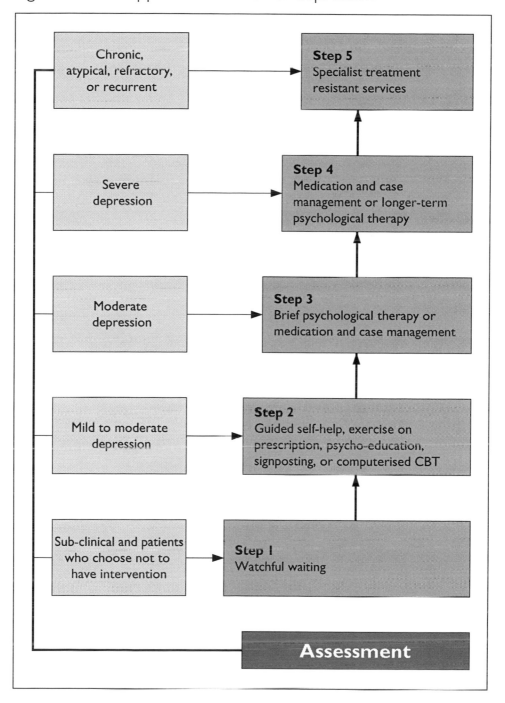

Stepped care is a model of healthcare delivery originating from the US, which has been applied to a range of psychological disorders. There are two key principles in the stepped care system. First, the recommended treatment should be the least intensive of those currently available, but still likely to provide significant health gain. For example, cognitive behaviour therapy (CBT) is a psychological treatment strongly recommended by the Department of Health (2001a) for anxiety and depression. CBT is traditionally delivered by a trained CBT therapist and is an intensive and expensive treatment; access to it is limited in primary care. Using a stepped care framework, it is feasible to offer CBT treatments in the first instance by using self-help approaches supported by brief contacts with a mental health worker with less advanced CBT training.

The second key principle of the stepped care model is that treatments and treatment outcomes are monitored systematically, and changes are made where indicated: by stepping 'up' to more intensive treatment if patient's condition is not improving, or 'down' to less intensive treatment if it is.

Steps 1-3 of the stepped care model involve treatment of patients in primary care and a key challenge has been how to implement these steps. Clinical pathways for depression have been developed to help with implementation (see Fletcher *et al*, 2004).

In addition, the government provided some support for primary mental health care in the NHS Plan (Department of Health, 2000), which promised by 2004 one thousand new 'graduate primary care mental health workers' trained in brief therapy techniques to help GPs manage and treat common mental health problems. These new workers were to assist primary care in the treatment of patients with common mental health problems by delivering brief psychological interventions, help audit activity and outcomes, and network with other organisations within the local community, especially with the voluntary sector and self-help support groups.

Improving access to psychological therapies is currently high on the political agenda. Economist Richard Layard (2006) has attracted considerable government interest with his argument that increased provision of psychological therapies (especially CBT) will help reduce the number of people rendered economically inactive and reliant on long-term incapacity benefits through depression and common mental disorders. Mental health problems account for a significant number of days lost from work and a significant proportion of patients on incapacity benefits. If psychological therapy can support return to work, the costs of providing a national workforce of psychological therapists can be recouped through reduced benefit payments and increased productivity, he argues.

Despite the high prevalence of mental health problems in primary care and positive changes in government policy, many patients' mental health problems go unrecognised, and therefore untreated. The Department of Health has sought to encourage better identification and treatment of common mental disorders in primary care. For example, the quality and outcomes (QOF) framework of the national GP contract offers practices additional payments for delivering specific clinical outcomes in a number of clinical domains (NHS Confederation, 2003). Depression outcomes have been a recent addition to QOF, which states:

- GPs are to routinely screen for depression in high risk groups such as patients with diabetes and coronary heart disease

- patients with a new diagnosis of depression are to have an assessment of severity at the outset of treatment using an assessment tool validated for use in primary care.

Practices can choose not to implement QOF, although it is envisaged most will be persuaded by the financial rewards attached to it.

Interventions

There has been an upsurge in activity in primary care to address mental health issues. New initiatives have introduced improvements in the workforce and supported new ways of thinking about clinical interventions. When treatment other than medication is indicated or requested by the patient, there are now several options available, many of which have a strong evidence base. However, despite these promising developments, variations in local resources mean that access to the full range of possible treatments remains patchy. The main options are detailed below.

Watchful waiting

According to the NICE guidance (2004a), watchful waiting can be used with patients who do not want treatment and those whom the health professional thinks will recover without intervention. Typically, this means reviewing the patient two weeks after the initial presentation and negotiating either further routine follow-up by the GP or, if there is no improvement or worsening of symptoms, stepping up to a higher level of intervention within the stepped care model. The GP will also provide the patient with written information on depression and treatments.

Exercise on prescription (EoP)

Being physically active can assist in the recovery of depression and anxiety and can also prevent against re-occurrence. However, seven in ten adults are not active enough to get the health benefits. EoP government schemes aim to tackle health inequalities by improving access to sport and exercise for those patients who cannot otherwise afford to participate. EoP can be used as a non-drug treatment for common mental health problems and aims to help people increase their physical activity. Many of the schemes already in operation have established links with local leisure centres and patients can access the equipment and receive regular advice and monitoring from qualified registered fitness professionals. National standards for EoP have been published by the Department of Health (2001b), which has encouraged the development of new and effective high quality projects nationwide.

An extension of these principles to leisure and education activities more broadly and to social support has been explored by some practices (SEU, 2004; Friedli & Watson, 2004).

Group psycho-education

This approach can be used in a range of non-healthcare environments, including health and adult education settings. Group psycho-education for mild depression and anxiety involves providing information about common mental health problems, issues that affect mood, how to identify and change thoughts, activities and interactions that affect mood, plus relaxation training and goal planning. Groups of six to ten people are formed locally and each group meets for eight sessions of up to two hours. It can be used as a preventive intervention (ie. with patients at risk of developing depression) or with patients presenting with specific symptoms of anxiety or depression such as panic or agoraphobia.

Referral facilitation ('signposting')

Referral facilitation involves a professional assessing a patient and assisting them to find help from other services, including self-help organisations and voluntary sector providers. This approach is dependent on the availability of local groups, up-to-date information on what they offer, and agreement from these groups concerning referral. Liaison with such groups and organisations is part of the envisaged role of the graduate mental health worker. Referral facilitation is appropriate for mental health problems of mild to moderate severity, and may be suitable for patients with depressive symptoms who are facing particular psychosocial difficulties for which there are relevant groups available.

Guided self-help

Guided self-help is appropriate for mild to moderate anxiety and depression. Self-help involves providing patients with both information about a condition and also skills and techniques to overcome symptoms and assist with problems. These skills and techniques are often based on CBT principles and techniques, which the patient can learn from books or computer programmes, supported by brief, regular, face-to-face contact with a primary health care practitioner to provide encouragement to use the materials and monitor outcome. Some computerised packages are designed to function with very little guidance, although monitoring of outcomes is still recommended. There is some evidence from the UK that 'pure self-help' using written materials improves outcomes for patients with depression in primary care, and that guided self-help can be conducted by non-mental health specialists such as practice nurses (Richards *et al*, 2002).

Brief cognitive behaviour therapy

CBT aims to help people address how they think – about themselves, the world, other people – and understand that how they behave affects their thoughts and feelings. Unlike most talking treatments, the focus is primarily on the here and now, rather than the roots or causes of the distress. The health professional and patient develop a shared understanding of the individual's problem and together identify goals and strategies for changing their ways of thinking and behaviours, which they monitor and evaluate over the course of treatment. CBT has proven effectiveness for a wide variety of psychological problems including anxiety and depression. Traditionally, 'full' CBT is delivered in one-hour weekly appointments over a 16-24 week period. However, 'brief' CBT of just six one-hour weekly appointments has been shown to be effective and to improve access to talking treatments when delivered in primary care (Churchill *et al*, 2001).

Computerised CBT

Computerised CBT (CCBT) involves the delivery of CBT using an interactive computer interface. Several CCBT packages are currently available, specific to different disorders. These packages require minimal facilitation and administrative support although access to a computer and a password to enter the system is required, and a licence fee must be paid, which can be a considerable cost to primary care trusts. NICE (2006) has recently reviewed their guidance on the use of CCBT in routine clinical practice, including recommendations on the most effective computerised packages for treating mild to moderate depression and panic and phobia.

Collaborative care and case management

Collaborative care introduces 'case managers' to the primary care team. These are health professionals with less intensive mental health training than specialists who work with patients and liaise closely with the GP and the mental health specialist. Case managers are based in the GP practice and take responsibility for proactively following up patients, assessing patient adherence to psychological and pharmacological treatments, delivering psychological support, monitoring patient progress and initiating further action when treatment is unsuccessful.

Books on prescription

The idea of providing self-help books by prescription (bibliotherapy) began in Cardiff in 2003 as a joint venture between local primary care services and local libraries. GPs and other primary care professionals are provided with a list of recommended self-help books and a 'book' prescription pad. The pad is used to 'prescribe' a particular book for a patient who can then borrow the book 'on prescription' from the local library. The books prescribed are often informed by CBT principles. Initial outcomes have been positive (eg. Reeves & Stace, 2005), and many more GP practices have adopted the idea.

Welfare and benefit advisors

Millions of people are living in poverty in the UK, many of whom are unemployed and not claiming the social security benefits to which they are entitled. People with mental health problems are particularly vulnerable. The availability of welfare rights advice in primary care has been shown to lead to significant financial and non-financial gains (Nuffield Institute for Health, 2002), and has been proposed as an intervention with significant potential to reduce inequalities in health.

Implementation issues

As noted previously, there have been a number of developments in improving primary care mental health services. However further work is required if the recommendations are to be implemented and targets achieved.

The development of the primary care graduate mental health worker role has seen an increase in the availability of treatments and the numbers of patients treated with psychological interventions in primary care (Fletcher *et al*, 2006). However, many areas have struggled to implement the role, often because there are insufficient resources or motivation to provide leadership, supervision and management in primary care. In addition, where recruitment has been successful, many workers have left the job in the first year or two, partly because of the lack of a career structure. In order to make the graduate worker role a viable and sustainable part of the workforce, these problems will have to be addressed. In addition, few designated posts currently exist for GPs with a special interest in mental health – a role that could significantly aid the primary care sector to manage the high volume of patients presenting with complex psychosocial problems.

While the economic arguments for expanding access to psychological therapies has been powerfully made (Layard, 2006), the numbers of therapists said to be required (10,000, half of them qualified clinical psychologists and the other drawn from a range of other healthcare professions) presents a major challenge in terms of training and recruitment. There are doubts as to whether primary care really needs such a large number of highly skilled CBT therapists, when the job might be done as effectively by less well qualified professionals.

Future commissioning developments may further change the way primary care mental health services are delivered. Practice based commissioning (PBC), for example, may bring access to a wider choice of treatments in primary care as it enables GPs to commission care and other services directly from provider organisations. This could mean flexibility to provide individually tailored packages drawing on local practitioners and providers, rather than having to use those with whom the primary care trust has negotiated a block contract.

Primary care responses to mental health have improved considerably in the last five years and we need to build on the success, providing faster access to effective treatments to a much wider group of clients, and providing it earlier to prevent illness from becoming chronic. If we aim to empower people to control their own lives, then increasing the availability of brief interventions has to be an important option.

References

British Medical Association (2003) *National enhanced service: specialised care of patients with depression.* London: BMA. (www.bma.org.uk/ap.nsf/Content/NESdepression)

Churchill R, Hunot V, Corney R *et al* (2001) A systematic review of controlled trials of the effectiveness and cost-effectiveness of brief psychological treatments for depression. *Health Technology Assessment* **5** (35).

Department of Health (1999) *National service framework for mental health: modern standards and service models.* London: the Stationery Office.

Department of Health (2000) *The NHS plan: a plan for investment; a plan for reform.* London: The Stationery Office.

Department of Health (2001a) *Treatment choice in psychological therapies and counselling: evidence based clinical practice guideline.* London. Department of Health.

Department of Health (2001b) *Exercise referral systems: a national quality assessment framework.* London: Department of Health.

Fletcher J, Bower P, Richards D *et al* (2004) *Enhanced services specification for depression under the new GP contract – a commissioning guidebook.* Manchester: NIMHE North West Regional Development Centre.

Fletcher J, Gask L, Robinson J *et al* (2006) *Primary care mental health collaborative.* Manchester: NIMHE North West Regional Development Centre.

Friedli L, Watson S (2004) *Social prescribing for mental health.* York: Northern Centre for Mental Health.

Gask L, Rogers A, Roland M *et al* (2003) *A practical guide to the national service framework for mental health.* London: National Primary Care Research and Development Centre.

Goldberg D, Huxley P (1992) *Common mental disorders: a biosocial model.* London: Routledge.

Kupfer DJ (1991) Long-term treatment of depression. *Journal of Clinical Psychiatry* **52** (s5) 28-34.

Layard R (2006) *The depression report: a new deal for depression and anxiety disorders.* London Centre for Economic Performance, London School of Economics. (http://cep.lse.ac.uk)

Lovell K, Richards D (2000) Multiple access points and levels of entry (MAPLE): ensuring choice, accessibility and equity for CBT services. *Behaviour and Cognitive Psychotherapy* **28** 379-391.

Murray CJ, Lopez AD (1996) *The global burden of disease: a comprehensive assessment of mortality and disability from diseases, injuries and risk factors in 1990 and projected to 2020 vol 1.* Cambridge, Mass: Harvard School of Public Health on behalf of the World Health Organization and the World Bank.

NHS Confederation (2003) *New GMS contract 2003: investing in general practice.* London: NHS Confederation.

NHS Confederation (2005) Adult mental health services in primary care. *Leading Edge* **17**.

NICE (2004a) *Depression: the management of depression in primary and secondary care.* London: NICE.

NICE (2004b) *Anxiety: management of anxiety (panic disorder, with or without agoraphobia, and generalised anxiety disorder) in adults in primary, secondary and community care.* London: NICE.

NICE (2006) *Depression and anxiety: computerised cognitive behavioural therapy (CCBT).* Technology appraisal. London: NICE.

Nuffield Institute for Health (2002) *Welfare advice in primary care.* London: Nuffield Institute for Health.

Reeves T, Stace JM (2005) Improving patient access and choice: assisted bibliotherapy for mild to moderate stress/anxiety in primary care. *Journal of Psychiatric Mental Health Nursing* **12** (3) 341-346.

Richards D, Richards A, Barkham M *et al* (2002) PHASE: a 'health technology' approach to psychological treatment in primary mental health care. *Primary Health Care Research and Development* **3** 159-168.

Sartorius N (2001) The economic and social burden of depression. *Journal of Clinical Psychiatry* **62** (s15) 8-11.

Simon GE, Goldberg DP, von Korff M (2002) Understanding cross-national differences in depression prevalence. *Psychological Medicine* **32** (4) 585-594.

Social Exclusion Unit (2004) *Mental health and social inclusion.* London: ODPM.

Chapter 13
Closing the gap: tackling physical health inequalities in primary care

Andrew Nocon and Liz Sayce

People with a serious mental health problem are twice as likely as the rest of the population to die prematurely (Harris & Barraclough, 1998). Even when deaths from unnatural causes such as suicide are taken into account, their mortality rate remains significantly higher.

Some of this is related to the greater prevalence of smoking-related fatal disease among people with schizophrenia (Joukamaa *et al*, 2001), including an increased risk of arteriosclerosis and sudden cardiac death (Davidson, 2002). Diabetes, too, is more common among people with schizophrenia (Mukherjee *et al*, 1996). The links between depression and physical illness are also becoming increasingly well known: having depression as well as a physical illness can worsen the prognosis for both (Barth *et al*, 2005).

These facts – all well-established in the literature – prompted the Disability Rights Commission (DRC) in December 2004 to launch an 18-month investigation, entitled Health Inequalities: Closing the Gap, into the health inequalities experienced by people with mental health problems and/or learning disabilities in England and Wales. The aim was to understand these inequalities, their causes, the extent to which recent initiatives have or have not helped to address the problems, what remains to be done, and how measures can be effectively implemented to prevent unnecessary ill-health or death.

The investigation included consultation with over 1000 people with mental health problems or learning disabilities, analysis of eight million primary care records (probably the most comprehensive study of primary care and mental health records in the world), detailed area studies in four areas, reviews of evidence of effective practice, and an inquiry panel that took written and oral evidence to establish achievable recommendations.

Findings

The primary care records analysis showed that:

- people with schizophrenia or bipolar disorder are more than twice as likely (2.4 times) as the rest of the population to have diabetes.

They are also:

- 1.6 times more likely to have ischaemic heart disease
- 1.8 times more likely to have stroke
- 1.3 times more likely to have hypertension.

In addition, it found that:

- people with schizophrenia are 1.9 times more likely to have bowel cancer – the second most common cause of cancer death in the UK
- women with schizophrenia are 1.4 times more likely to have breast cancer.

People with depression, too, are:

- 1.6 times more likely than people without mental health problems to have ischaemic heart disease
- 1.8 times more likely to have a stroke
- 1.5 times more likely to have diabetes
- 1.6 times more likely to have chronic obstructive airways disease.

Rates of obesity and smoking are high:

- 33% of people with schizophrenia and 30% of people with bipolar disorder are obese, compared with 21% in the rest of the population

- 61% of people with schizophrenia and 46% of people with bipolar disorder smoke, compared with 33% of the general population (where smoking status was recorded).

Both these factors put them at greater risk of serious health problems and early death.

Not only are people with major mental health problems more likely than other citizens to develop some significant health problems; they are likely to develop them at a younger age. By the age of 55:

- 31% of people with schizophrenia have coronary heart disease (CHD)
- 41% have diabetes
- 21% have suffered a stroke
- 23% have serious respiratory disease.

The figures for the general population are 18%, 30%, 11% and 17% respectively.

Once they have developed these conditions, they are likely to die sooner than other people. Adjusting for age, the percentages of people with schizophrenia who have died from these conditions after five years are:

- 22% of people with CHD
- 19% of people with diabetes
- 28% of people who have had a stroke
- 28% of people with respiratory disease.

The comparable percentages for people with no serious mental health problems are all lower, at 8%, 9%, 12% and 15% respectively. For people with bipolar disorder with those conditions, the figures are 15%, 4%, 19% and 24%.

Although deprivation is a key determinant of poor health and mortality, and people with mental health problems are more likely to live in deprived circumstances, not all the differences in health can be attributed to social deprivation.

Using primary care services

Accessing health assessments and treatment can be a major problem. We know that some people with mental health problems are not registered with a GP. They may have been struck off and have experienced problems finding another GP; it can be difficult for people to 'clear their name' or obtain redress if it has been alleged by a professional that they are aggressive or 'difficult'. Obtaining permanent registration with a GP can be particularly difficult for refugees, asylum-seekers and homeless people. People told us:

'I have been removed from GPs' lists as "too demanding" and told off the record my needs are too expensive.'

'I was removed from the panel because I made a complaint about inaccurate records and neglect.'

Experiences of primary healthcare are very variable. Many people speak highly of the services they receive, but others report inappropriate stereotyping, negative attitudes and detrimental assumptions about the quality of life a person with mental health problems can expect. While these attitudes may not always be associated with poorer outcomes, they do reflect the extent to which people's concerns are taken seriously or dismissed, and whether symptoms are explored and opportunities to carry out screening or reviews of medication are taken up. We were told:

'The receptionist has a bad attitude because of my mental health problems and I find them rude at times.'

'They exacerbate my condition, by being generally shunning of disability, being discriminatory, bullying, neglectful, unconfident, accusing – generally outrageously unprofessional and even suggesting I am not worthy of support as I can offer nothing to society.'

One of the most common problems is 'diagnostic overshadowing', with physical health problems being wrongly attributed to the mental health condition:

'The doctor just assumes that everything is psychological. If he can't find a reason for it with just talking to me, then it can't be a real illness.'

'My GP seems to think that everything I go to him for is related to my mental health impairment. So much so that he first told me a lump I found was not there until I pushed for a second opinion, whereby a tumour the size of an orange was found.'

Negative attitudes and a lack of serious attention to problems mean that people may be put off from contacting a doctor when they need to:

'She makes me feel I am doing wrong by not being well enough to work and from many of her comments to me she does not believe I am telling the truth. Because of this undermining attitude I very rarely feel able to go to my GP, even if I am very unwell.'

'I hate going to see him, it makes me so anxious because of that awful wariness that he seems to have, as if I am a leper and might do something unexpected at any minute… It just hurts to see how people are so wary.'

Fear and mistrust can work in both directions. As the report on the area studies put it:

'The subtext from the interviews with primary care staff and practitioners was a mix of fear, anxiety and some impatience combined with paternalism and kindness. Even though some of the interviews described the provision of awareness training in both mental health and learning difficulty, there was still a sense that patients from these groups were like time bombs ready to go off at any moment.'

Some practitioners' attitudes were praised, particularly where they themselves had personal or family experience of mental health problems. Evidence suggests that attitudes shift through personal experience – or contact with someone with a mental health problem, on equal terms. This has implications for mental health service user involvement in leadership, employment and training.

We also noted a considerable difference between the views of primary care practitioners and service users about the effectiveness of services. While practitioners felt that they were providing as good a service as possible, and viewed access problems as stemming from the individual's condition or chaotic lifestyle, service users thought that services could be considerably improved and that responsibility for access problems lay with the services.

Health promotion

The types of health problems that people with severe mental illness experience mean there is a key role for health promotion. We know from other research that smoking cessation advice, blood pressure checks or prescriptions for exercise are often lacking. We wanted to know whether people with mental health problems get the same levels of service as everyone else. Some findings are encouraging. People with long-term mental health problems who smoke, for instance, are slightly more likely to receive smoking cessation advice and be prescribed smoking cessation medication (65% and 10% compared with 59% and 8% among smokers in the general population).

However, these quantitative findings tell us nothing about the quality of the advice: it may be that the higher rate simply reflects higher consultation rates and GPs using the opportunity to mention smoking cessation. Also, people with mental health problems are more likely than the general population to be on low incomes and so to be entitled to free prescriptions for medication.

Practitioners who responded to our consultation questionnaire were cynical about the effectiveness of health promotion. One view was that smoking cessation programmes generally do not work for people with mental health problems – even though the evidence indicates that they do, albeit with lower quit rates than in the general population (Samele *et al*, 2006; Doherty, 2006). This lack of enthusiasm is likely to translate into health promotion advice being near the bottom of the priority list in consultations. Of the 69 people with mental health problems who took part in focus groups or interviews in the area studies, only a minority had received health promotion advice from primary healthcare staff. With low levels of active or targeted help to quit (as opposed to simple advice), coupled with low expectations, it is unlikely that the scale of the challenge of high smoking rates can be effectively met.

Tests and treatment

Compared with the general population with the same physical health problems, we found that:

- people with schizophrenia and ischaemic heart disease were less likely to have had a blood pressure reading in the previous 15 months, and less likely to have had a recent cholesterol test

- people with schizophrenia and stroke were less likely to have had a cholesterol test in the past 15 months, and less likely to be taking aspirin as a preventive measure (63%, compared to 68% among other people who had had a stroke)

- 66% of people with schizophrenia who also have CHD were likely to be prescribed statins to reduce lipids (fats) in the blood, compared with 81% in the case of other people with CHD

- only 63% of eligible women with schizophrenia had had a cervical smear in the previous five years, compared with 73% of women in the rest of the population.

Including mental health indicators in the quality and outcomes framework of the new General Medical Services contract may have helped to increase the extent to which physical health checks are provided for people with serious mental health problems. According to an analysis of the first year's contract data undertaken for our investigation, 76% of practices reported that they had carried out reviews in the preceding 15 months for at least 90% of registered patients with severe long-term mental health problems, and 40% said they had reviewed every such patient on their register. Although guidance has been provided about the content of these reviews, we do not know what they have actually involved. It is notable that the data on lower levels of prescription of statins for people with schizophrenia and CHD were from the first full year of the new contract: the checks in their current form are clearly not enough.

More encouragingly, though, we found that a higher proportion of people with serious mental health problems had had their blood pressure recorded over the past five years compared with the remaining population, and more people with schizophrenia had a normal blood pressure reading. And there were no differences in the investigations people received following postmenopausal or rectal bleeding, both of which can be symptoms of cancer.

Side effects of medication

Psychotropic medication is known to have a serious adverse impact on physical health and mortality rates. A number of psychotropic drugs are associated with cardiac side effects; these are particularly likely to be serious where there is coexistent mild heart disease (Witchel *et al*, 2003). Adverse interactions between general medical and psychotropic drugs are well established, including both antipsychotics and antidepressants (Goldman, 2000; Bingefors *et al*, 1996). Antidepressant treatment is itself a predictor of increased mortality in older people, notably from cardiovascular causes and even when controlling for pre-existing chronic medical disease (Bingefors *et al*, 1996). The concurrent prescription of more than one antipsychotic is also associated with reduced survival (Joukamaa *et al*, 2006).

The major weight gain induced by antipsychotics represents a serious concern. In addition, psychotropic and antidepressant medication can cause cardiovascular disease, hypotension, impaired glucose tolerance and increased prolactin levels (associated with decreased bone mineral density, infertility and amenorrhoea) (Scanlan & Houltram, undated). NICE guidance on schizophrenia recommends that GPs should discuss the benefits and side-effects of medication before it is prescribed (NICE, 2002). Medication monitoring and review is particularly important for older people, who are more likely to be taking a number of medicines and to be more sensitive to their effects. In practice, however, the management of side effects can leave a lot to be desired. We were told:

'My GP is very good in the way of listening but like most GPs does not warn patients of side effects if put onto new drugs. Has lots of literature on diabetes, stroke, heart problems but nothing in relation to mental health or neurological problems like epilepsy, which I feel are all very closely linked.'

'I am dismayed and surprised that my consultant psychiatrist has advised me to remain permanently on antidepressants. I have been taking this drug for six years (with unpleasant physical side effects). He has never suggested that an alternative antidepressant may be a better option. It is my experience that some psychiatrists are oblivious to the negative response in the elderly to certain drugs. I feel I am living in a permanent fog – simply existing and not living.'

Healthcare for people from BME communities

Little evidence is currently available about the physical healthcare needs of people from black and minority ethnic (BME) communities who have mental health problems, although work is being initiated in some parts of the country to identify and address them. However, the reluctance of some people from some BME communities to contact primary care services about mental health problems, resulting from their adverse experiences of mental health services, coupled with data from a national census showing they are more likely to be referred to specialist mental health services via the criminal justice system rather than primary care (Healthcare Commission, 2005), gives cause for concern and highlights the importance of paying particular attention to their physical health needs.

People in inpatient settings

People in inpatient psychiatric settings rarely have any contact with primary care. In one instance where a primary care service was provided, demand outstripped supply and access to the service had to be curtailed (Welthagen et al, 2004).

What needs to be done

Although the problems are widespread, there are also many examples of good practice. These are frequently at practice level, such as appointments being easy to arrange, helpful attitudes, and doctors who listen. Addressing physical health issues also requires good working relationships between primary care teams, psychiatrists and community mental health teams. The Royal College of Psychiatrists has prepared a set of recommendations to ensure that psychiatrists monitor and address the physical health issues relating to mental healthcare. Physical health checks are supposed to be included in assessments under the Care Programme Approach (CPA) and care plans should identify physical health needs. However, the extent to which the CPA is used to assess physical health needs is very variable. In some areas, checks are only offered to people on enhanced CPA. Resource constraints are one reason why checks are not provided more widely.

The Department of Health has published guidance for PCTs on commissioning physical health care services for people with severe, long-term mental health problems, which includes several examples of best practice (Department of Health, 2006). It has also funded 88 'spearhead' PCTs to employ specialist nurses to improve access to physical health care services for people with severe mental illness. Other examples of good practice can be found among the shortlisted entries to the NIMHE positive practice awards: for example, the 2005 entries included a sport and exercise project, a network of service users and workers involved in physical activities, and a collaborative project between an assertive outreach team and primary care that helps users to access physical health services and improve their lifestyles (NIMHE, 2005).

The DRC's final report (DRC, 2006) makes a number of recommendations for mental health and primary care providers (*Table 1*). The full report also includes further detailed recommendations for commissioners, performance management and inspection bodies, standard-setting and good practice organisations, and government. The new Disability Equality Duty[1] provides a key framework for taking the recommendations forward. Putting the recommendations into practice is essential if poor physical health and early deaths are to be effectively addressed.

Perhaps most importantly, the historically low expectations that people with mental health problems 'just do' die younger need to be tackled, by government and health professionals, and by mental health service users themselves by knowing and asserting their rights.

The full report Equal Treatment: Closing the Gap *can be downloaded from www.drc.org.uk*

---

[1] See www.drc.org.uk/employers_and_service_provider/disability_equality_duty.aspx

Table 1: Recommendations

Mental health service providers

- Minimise and monitor the adverse effects of psychiatric medication, and revise medication accordingly. Inform people of benefits and risks – including risks to physical health – so that service users can decide on the trade-off between relief of psychiatric symptoms and physical side-effects.

- Ensure through care plans that service users can access primary care to quality and outcome framework standards.

- Include inreach primary care services in contracts for inpatient psychiatric units.

- Positively promote healthy living, both for people living in the community and in inpatient settings. This will include:
  - providing smoking cessation advice, support and interventions
  - advice and support with weight management
  - encouragement and support to take exercise
  - promoting a healthy environment, where people have easy access to a healthy diet and exercise and live smoke-free.

- Support to ensure that physical health needs are appropriately addressed within primary care.

Primary health care providers

- Establish mandatory training for primary care staff, to counteract diagnostic overshadowing and improve attitudes and understanding.

- Offer people with mental health problems the option of recording their access needs – and then make provision to meet them as essential requirements under the Disability Discrimination Act. These could include different appointment lengths, choice of early or late appointments to avoid queuing, text or telephone appointment reminders, telephone consultations, or specific waiting arrangements.

- Minimise and monitor adverse effects of psychiatric medication, and revise medication accordingly. Ensure people understand treatment options and can make active choices.

- Offer regular evidence-based health checks.

- Ensure people receive any health promotion, screening and physical treatment they require.

- Ensure that, in line with the GMS contract and BMA guidance, no one is removed from or refused access to a GP list because of their mental health problems.

- Make direct contact with local mental health groups and involve them in advising on improvements to the experience of using primary care and in auditing services and delivering training to the whole primary care team.

References

Barth J, Schumacher M, Herrmann-Lingen C (2005) Depression as a risk factor for mortality in patients with coronary heart disease: a meta-analysis. *Psychosomatic Medicine* **66** (6) 802-813.

Bingefors K, Isacson D, von Knorring L *et al* (1996) Antidepressant-treated patients in ambulatory care: mortality during a nine-year period after first treatment. *British Journal of Psychiatry* **169** (5) 647-654.

Davidson M (2002) Risk of cardiovascular disease and sudden death in schizophrenia. *Journal of Clinical Psychiatry* **63** (s9) 5-11.

Department of Health (2006) *Choosing health: supporting the physical needs of people with severe mental illness - commissioning framework.* London: Department of Health.

Disability Rights Commission (2006) *Equal treatment: closing the gap.* London: Disability Rights Commission.

Doherty K (2006) Giving up the habit. *Mental Health Today* (May) 27-29.

Goldman LS (2000) Comorbid medical illness in psychiatric patients. *Current Psychiatry Reports* **2** 256-263.

Harris SC, Barraclough B (1998) Excess mortality of mental disorder. *British Journal of Psychiatry* **173** 11-53.

Healthcare Commission (2005) *Count me in: results of a national census of inpatients in mental health hospitals and facilities in England and Wales.* London: Healthcare Commission.

Joukamaa M, Heliovaara M, Knekt P *et al* (2001) Mental disorders and cause-specific mortality. *British Journal of Psychiatry* **179** 498-502.

Joukamaa M, Heliovaara M, Knekt P *et al* (2006) Schizophrenia, neuroleptic medication and mortality. *British Journal of Psychiatry* **188** 122-127.

Mukherjee S, Decina P, Bocola V *et al* (1996) Diabetes mellitus in schizophrenic patients. *Comprehensive Psychiatry* **37** (1) 68-73.

National Institute for Clinical Excellence (2002) *Core interventions in the treatment and management of schizophrenia in primary and secondary care.* London: NICE.

National Institute for Mental Health (England) (2004a) *Physical health needs of people with mental health problems: guidance for health and social care professionals.* Leeds: NIMHE.

National Institute for Mental Health (England) (2004b) *What you can expect. Physical health needs of people with mental health problems: guidance for mental health service users.* Leeds: NIMHE.

National Institute for Mental Health (England) (2005) *Positive practice awards 2005.* (http://nimhe.csip.org.uk/index.cfm?fuseaction=main.viewItem&intItemID=80717)

Samele C, Hoadley A, Seymour L (2006) *A systematic review of the effectiveness of interventions to improve the physical health of people with severe mental health problems.* London: Disability Rights Commission.

Scanlan M, Houltram B (undated). *A care map for the assessment and management of atypical antipsychotic side effects.* Northampton: Centre for Healthcare Education, University College Northampton. (www.primhe.org/live/webroot/files/AstZen-Care%20Map.pdf)

Welthagen E, Talbot S, Harrison O *et al* (2004) Providing a primary care service for psychiatric in-patients. *Psychiatric Bulletin* **28** 167-170.

Witchel HJ, Hancox JC, Nutt DJ (2003) Psychotropic drugs, cardiac arrhythmia and sudden death. *Journal of Clinical Psychopharmacology* **23** (1) 58-77.

Chapter 14
Risk management in mental health: people, perceptions and places

Tony Ryan

Societies have been concerned since time immemorial about the threats that people with mental health problems pose to others (Foucault, 1971). The risk that such people pose to themselves has tended almost invariably to be a secondary concern. Here in the UK such concerns have been heightened in the past two decades by a series of high profile homicides with their attendant public inquiries and recommendations, all coming to very similar conclusions and all, seemingly, making little difference.

Risk in mental health has been largely understood in negative terms, as synonymous with danger, threat and adverse events. However, in other areas of life risks are positively sought after for the potential rewards they can bring: for example, people risk a few pounds gambling on the National Lottery, or indeed risk their own lives by driving fast or taking up an extreme sport like sky diving. In such a context, risk-taking may even be seen as laudable.

Unfortunately media coverage of the rare adverse events that occur in the mental health context has led to defensive practice on the part of mental health professionals, providers and policy makers. This is to be expected, to some degree, particularly when there is a strong imperative to demonstrate learning from what went wrong in other instances. But such a climate can discourage positive risk taking: that is, taking risks with a positive, empowering or therapeutic purpose. Happily this is now recognised (Bassett *et al*, 2005). That said, during the early stages of a mental health problem it can be difficult (although not impossible) to take positive risks. It could even be argued that one of the greatest risks that people face is not getting effective treatment soon enough (Ho *et al*, 2003). However, once this 'acute' stage has passed, the process of recovery has to involve risk taking (Repper & Perkins, 2003): indeed, it is an essential part of the recovery process. Nevertheless, this can go very much against the culture that prevails in mental health services.

What are the risks?
Harm to others
A small number of homicides are committed each year by people who have been in recent contact with mental health services. These numbers have decreased steadily

from 35% of all homicides in 1957 to 11.5% in 1995 (Taylor & Gunn, 1999). By 1997-2000 just nine per cent of homicides in England and Wales were committed by people who had been in contact with mental health services in the year before the offence (Appleby *et al*, 2001). Moreover, not all of these people would necessarily have been mentally ill at the time of the offence, and only 20% of those who did have symptoms of mental illness at the time of the offence had had contact with the mental health services in the previous 12 months. The mistaken public perception that such homicides have been occurring more frequently in recent years (in fact they have been declining by a steady three per cent since 1957) is arguably due more to the negative publicity attached to such events by the media than to anything else (Paterson, 2006). On the other hand, the reforms in mental health service provision introduced in recent years would seem to have had no impact to date in reducing such homicides.

Suicide

Suicides by people in recent contact with mental health services account for approximately 28% of all recorded suicides and open verdicts (CSIP, 2006). The national strategy for suicide prevention in England was launched in 2002 (Department of Health, 2002) and its report for the year 2005 suggests a slight fall in the overall suicide rate in England since that date (CSIP, 2006).

Self-harm

The risk of self-harm in relation to mental illness is somewhat misunderstood, particularly by health and social care professionals who do not have specialist knowledge of the field. On the one hand there is some evidence that people who self harm are at a higher risk of suicide (Hawton & van Heeringen, 2002). On the other hand, there is a growing body of evidence that for many people self-harm is itself a coping (risk management) strategy, and is not always synonymous with an intent to die (Shaw & Hogg, 2004; Ryan, 2000).

Self-neglect

This somewhat disparaging term has been used as a catch-all phrase for describing the impact of symptoms associated with some forms of schizophrenia and depressive illnesses (Brown *et al*, 1999). At its most extreme self-neglect can lead to death, but it can also lead to over-protection by mental health services and professionals, who can find it difficult to take risks with people who appear unable to meet their own basic needs.

Social exclusion

Stigma and lack of opportunity are two of the key features of social exclusion as experienced by people with mental health problems. There is significant evidence to suggest that mental ill health results in social exclusion and that being refused opportunities to take an active and meaningful part in society creates mental health problems (Social Exclusion Unit, 2004).

Disempowerment

Using mental health services can itself be a disabling experience, particularly if the use is long-term. The disempowerment of people in mental health services is an insidious process. Service users can be seen in the 'sick role' and treated as such, which reinforces their inability to take responsibility for themselves. In extreme circumstances, where users are seen as 'difficult' (for whatever reasons), it can lead to what has been termed malignant alienation (that is, a progressive deterioration in relationships with others, including loss of sympathy and support from mental health workers, who can construe behaviour as provocative, unreasonable, or over-dependent) (Watts & Morgan, 1994). Institutionalisation is another form of disempowerment and, while the Victorian institutions have now disappeared, it has been suggested that many mental health service users have since become no less institutionalised and dependent in community services (Priebe & Turner, 2003).

Many of the above risks are interlinked and cannot be managed in isolation. People often talk of 'holistic treatment', but the reality is that, to be holistic, treatments must address the stigmatising effects of mental illness with as much genuine attention as they address clinical symptoms.

Risk assessment

Assessment is a crucial part of the management of risk, irrespective of its type. Whose assessment is the more accurate has been the subject of considerable debate between service users, carers and professionals. Although the term 'user involvement' has featured in almost every national policy document for the past two decades, in practice such involvement has not uniformly extended to risk assessment and risk management (Langan & Lindow 2004; Ryan, 2000).

Mental health professionals use three main methods to predict risk outcomes: clinical, actuarial and a combination of the two. Clinical risk assessment is often based on interviews with the person and/or some of the people in contact with them. Consequently, it involves a strong element of subjectivity and is susceptible to bias on the part of the clinician, who will be influenced by the models of mental health and treatment to which they subscribe and by past experiences.

Actuarial risk assessments use statistically derived population-based indicators to measure levels of risk. However, while this model may be useful as a broad-brush predictor of the likely behaviours of large numbers of people with similar risk factors, it tends not to be sufficiently sensitive to the idiosyncrasies of every individual they are used to assess.

The above methods of assessment are all professionally led. Service users and carers have argued for some time that their experiences and expertise can usefully inform the management of risk. Indeed, service users' strategies for assessment and management of their own risks have been shown to be extremely sophisticated

(Quirk *et al*, 2005; Ryan, 2002; Ryan, 2000), but use of this resource by professionals has been found to be very variable (Langan & Lindow, 2004).

Risk management

Risk is managed in mental health services through assessment, procedures and structures. The main formal procedure is the Care Programme Approach (NHS Executive & Social Services Inspectorate, 1999), which was explicitly introduced to provide a framework for risk management through care co-ordination. Failure adequately to implement the CPA and poor co-ordination of services have been cited as significant factors in numerous homicide and suicide inquiries (Warner, 2005). The use of CPA where independent sector services have been involved has also been found wanting and in need of improvement (Ryan *et al*, 2004). Moreover, while internal risk management structures within an organisation may be given significant attention (Healthcare Commission, 2004), where an individual's care involves discrete services provided by a range of different organisations there is considerably potential for failures to occur at the interconnection between the component parts.

Risk perceptions

One relatively unexplored area is perception of risk, and how this can affect the risk assessment and management processes. The service user's perspective can be very different to those of professionals and carers, and the perspectives of family and close friends can be different again. Very little research has been undertaken in relation to these differences and how a multifaceted understanding of risk from all these different perspectives might influence the quality and outcomes of its assessment and management. We do know, however, that gender is a significant variable in perceptions of mental health related risk (Ryan 1998). Irrespective of age, ethnicity, use of mental health services and whether the person is a professional, service user, carer or member of the public, women tend to rate risks of self-harm, harm to others, social exclusion and being disempowered by services higher than do men.

This is significant where risk assessment and management are concerned, as such perceptions will undoubtedly influence outcomes of assessments and consequent management decisions, and particularly so when clinical rather than actuarial judgements are made by the person carrying out the assessment. The obvious way to avoid the gender bias is to ensure that both men and women clinicians are involved in the assessment process. But an even more effective approach would be to ensure that service users and their significant others are genuinely involved in the process. Conflicts of interest can more easily be identified through this approach, making the decision-making more robust.

From risky people to risky places

Finally, much of the literature has been concerned with the risk that service users pose, whether to themselves or others. Thankfully, however, the emphasis is now broadening to examine both those who undertake risk assessment and management (Ryan, 1998; Gale *et al*, 2003) and the places where people are treated (Garcia *et al*, 2005; Quirk *et al*, 2005; Meehan *et al*, 2006). The focus on the risk assessor has made us aware not only of this gender influence on perceptions of risk but also that the assessor's understanding of probability in relation to risk outcomes can be somewhat limited (Gale *et al*, 2003).

In relation to inpatient services, a considerable body of evidence exists demonstrating that they can be very dangerous environments (Garcia *et al*, 2005; Healthcare Commission & Royal College of Psychiatrists, 2005), and that they do not offer adequate protection to some of the most vulnerable people in them (Meehan *et al*, 2006). Hearteningly, there is also a growing body of evidence demonstrating that service users have developed proactive strategies to manage risk in such places (Quirk *et al*, 2005; Ryan, 2000).

Conclusion

There is a considerable body of literature on risk and its management in mental health settings. There is also growing evidence to suggest that service users and carers have considerable risk management skills in their own right. National policy supports the need to balance risk management with user involvement, but overwhelmingly the experience of users and carers is that their own skills and resources are not being used to their full potential by mental health workers and organisations. I would argue that this is a wasted resource: that without such involvement, the management of risk in mental health will always be less than fully effective.

References

Appleby L, Shaw J, Sherratt J *et al* (2001) *Safety first: report of the National Confidential Inquiry into Suicide and Homicide by People with Mental Illness.* London: the Stationery Office.

Basset T, Lindley P, Barton R (2005) *The ten essential shared capabilities: a learning pack for mental health.* London: NHSU/NIMHE/Sainsbury Centre for Mental Health.

Brown S, Birtwistle J, Roe L *et al* (1999) The unhealthy lifestyle of people with schizophrenia. *Psychological Medicine* **29** (3) 697-701.

Care Services Improvement Partnership (2006) *National suicide prevention strategy for England – annual report on progress 2005.* Leeds: NIMHE.

Department of Health (1999) *National service framework for mental health: modern standards and service models.* London: Department of Health.

Department of Health (2000) *The NHS plan: a plan for investment, a plan for reform.* London: the Stationery Office.

Department of Health (2001) *Shifting the balance of power: securing delivery.* London: Department of Health.

Department of Health (2002) *Mental health policy implementation guide: community mental health teams.* London: Department of Health.

Foucault M (1971) *Madness and civilisation: a history of insanity in the age of reason.* London: Tavistock.

Gale T, Hawley C, Sivakumaran T (2003) Do mental health professionals really understand probability? Implications for risk assessment and evidence-based practice. *Journal of Mental Health* **12** (4) 417-430.

Gale T, Woodward A, Hawley C *et al* (2002) Risk assessment for people with mental health problems: a pilot study of reliability in working practice. *International Journal of Psychiatry in Clinical Practice* **6** (2) 73-81.

Garcia I, Kennett C, Quraishi M (2005) *Acute care 2004: a national survey of adult psychiatric wards in England.* London: Sainsbury Centre for Mental Health.

Hawton K, van Heeringen K (eds) (2002) *The international handbook of suicide and attempted suicide.* London: John Wiley & Sons.

Healthcare Commission (2004) *Framework for risk management: mental health trusts.* London: Healthcare Commission.

Healthcare Commission/Royal College of Psychiatrists (2005) *The national audit of violence (2003-2005): final report.* London: Healthcare Commission/Royal College of Psychiatrists.

Ho B-C, Alicata D, Ward J (2003) Untreated initial psychosis: relation to cognitive deficits and brain morphology in first-episode schizophrenia. *American Journal of Psychiatry* **160** 142-148.

Langan J, Lindow V (2004) *Living with risk: mental health service user involvement in risk assessment and management.* Bristol: The Policy Press.

Meehan J, Kapur N, Hunt I *et al* (2006) Suicide in mental health inpatients and within three months of discharge: national clinical survey. *British Journal of Psychiatry* **188** 129-134.

NHS Executive & Social Services Inspectorate (1999) *Effective care co-ordination in mental health services: modernising the care programme approach. A policy booklet.* London: NHSE/SSI.

Paterson B (2006) Newspaper representations of mental illness and the impact of the reporting of 'events' on social policy: the 'framing' of Isabel Schwarz and Jonathan Zito. *Journal of Psychiatric and Mental Health Nursing* **13** (3) 294-300.

Priebe S, Trevor T (2003) Reinstitutionalisation in mental health care. *British Medical Journal* **326** 175-176.

Quirk A, Lelliott P, Seale C (2005) Risk management by patients on psychiatric wards in London: an ethnographic study. *Health, Risk & Society* **7** (1) 85-91.

Repper J, Perkins R (2003) *Social inclusion and recovery: a model for mental health practice.* London: Bailliere Tindall.

Ryan T (1998) Perceived risks associated with mental illness: beyond homicide and suicide. *Social Science and Medicine* **46** (2) 287-297.

Ryan T (2000) Exploring the risk management strategies of mental health service users. *Health, Risk and Society* **2** (3) 267-282.

Ryan T (2002) Exploring the risk management strategies of informal carers of mental health service users. *Journal of Mental Health* **11** (1) 17-25.

Ryan T, Pearsall A, Hatfield B *et al* (2004) A pilot study of out of area placements for serious mental illness in the private sector. *Journal of Mental Health* **13** (4) 425-429.

Shaw C, Hogg C (2004) Shouting at the spaceman – a conversation about self-harm. In: Duffy D, Ryan T (eds) *New approaches to preventing suicide: a manual for practitioners.* London: Jessica Kingsley Publishers.

Social Exclusion Unit (2004) *Mental health and social exclusion.* London: Office of the Deputy Prime Minister.

Taylor P, Gunn J (1999) Homicides by people with mental illness: myth and reality. *British Journal of Psychiatry* **174** 9-14.

Warner L (2005) *Review of the literature on the Care Programme Approach.* London: Sainsbury Centre for Mental Health.

Watts D, Morgan G (1994) Malignant alienation: dangers for patients who are hard to like. *British Journal of Psychiatry* **164** (1) 11-15.

Chapter 15
Community mental health teams: a local whole systems approach

Steve Onyett

This chapter covers community teams for people with mental health problems, including community mental health teams (CMHTs, also sometimes called primary care liaison teams), early intervention teams, crisis resolution (also known as home treatment) teams (CRTs), and assertive outreach teams. Primary health care teams (even when they do not include any specialist mental health staff) also work with people with mental health problems and form an important part of how the whole local system of care works together effectively.

The CMHT configurations now in place are shaped by the mental health policy implementation guidance issued by the Department of Health in 2001 (Department of Health, 2001), building on the national service framework for mental health (NSF) (Department of Health, 1999), and the subsequent NHS Plan (Department of Health, 2000). In addition to the traditional CMHT model, we now have:

- assertive outreach teams. What distinguishes this approach is the intensity of engagement with clients in community settings in order to achieve effective working relationships with people who may be reluctant to have contact with mental health services. The model has its origins in assertive community treatment models, principally from the US (see Onyett, 2003)

- crisis resolution (or home treatment) teams. These provide a 24-hour service to users in community settings (normally at home) in order to avoid hospital admission wherever possible and provide the maximum opportunity to resolve crises in the contexts in which they occur

- early intervention teams. These also work proactively but specifically seek to engage with people in the early stages of developing psychotic symptoms. The aim is to reduce delay between onset of symptoms and access to services in order to improve outcomes and prevent long-term dependency on services (Birchwood *et al*, 1998)

This article will explore each of these team configurations before turning to some overarching issues. A thorough evaluation of the efficacy of these service models is beyond the scope of this article, but relevant signposting will be provided.

Community mental health teams

The community mental health team is regarded as 'the mainstay of the system' (Department of Health, 2002):

> 'CMHTs have an important, indeed integral, role to play in supporting service users and families in community settings. They should provide the core around which newer service elements are developed... They, alongside primary care, will provide the key source of referrals to the newer teams. They will also continue to care for the majority of people with mental illness in the community.' (Department of Health, 2002)

Guidance on CMHTs (Department of Health, 2002) states that the functions of the CMHT should be:

1 giving advice on the management of mental health problems by other professionals – in particular, advice to primary care and a triage function enabling appropriate referral

2 providing treatment and care for people with time-limited disorders who can benefit from specialist interventions

3 providing treatment and care for those with more complex and enduring needs.

Their main client group is intended to be people with 'time limited disorders [who can] be referred back to their GPs after a period of weeks or months'.

However the emerging picture from the field is one of conflicting demands, reduced resources, and lack of clarity about their role and function. Many CMHTs have continued to work with people with more complex health and social care needs (function 3 above), and in some cases have incorporated functions associated with early intervention and crisis work. A 2005 national survey of CRTs (Onyett *et al*, in preparation) found concerns over the lack of capacity in CMHTs to resume work with people following a period of crisis. The role of CMHTs in serving people with enduring and complex needs will also be influenced by the existence of local rehabilitation and recovery teams for people for who do not meet the eligibility criteria for assertive outreach. These teams are also described in the Department of Health's mental health policy implementation guide (MHPIG) (2001), but no targets were set for numbers to be available locally. In some cases they no longer exist and CMHTs have assumed their function, along with 'step down' care of clients referred from assertive outreach and crisis resolution teams.

Another stated function of CMHTs is to 'reduce stigma, [and] ensure that care is delivered in the least restrictive and disruptive manner possible'. It is questionable whether involvement with a designated mental health team is the least stigmatising way to provide care and support to individuals who might be better served through individual counselling, therapy, peer support or self-management provided in primary care.

Moreover, that specific targets were set for the number and capacities of the newer team approaches has often led to a fragmented approach to local development. Despite their supposed cornerstone status, the introduction of the new teams has in some cases meant that existing CMHTs have lost staff and status, while being expected to provide a default service for those clients whom the newer teams either fail to take on or refer back for step-down care. The existing services can therefore find themselves in a situation of increasing demand, with depleted capacity and reduced control over their workload (Burns, 2004).

In this confusing policy context, it is perhaps no surprise that CMHTs are the part of the local mental health system where there is least clarity and where the need for such teams at all is questioned. It is also that part of the local service system where practitioners may feel they have least control over their caseload: unlike the newer service models, they do not have recommended caseload sizes and clear eligibility criteria for admission to the team caseload. That, combined with potential role confusion, creates the optimal conditions for poor team and individual practitioner morale.

Despite these potentially adverse conditions the most recent mapping of services (see www.amhmapping.org.uk/reports) identifies 825 CMHTs nationally, compared with around 540 in 1993 (Onyett et al, 1994).

Assertive outreach teams

The National Forum for Assertive Outreach (NFAO, 2005) describes the key features of assertive outreach as follows:

- a discrete multidisciplinary team able to provide a full range of interventions

- most services provided directly by the team and not brokered out

- low staff to client ratios (1:10 to 1:15)

- most interventions provided in community settings

- emphasis on engagement and maintaining contact with clients

- caseloads shared across clinicians. Staff know and work with the entire caseload, although a Care Programme Approach (CPA) care co-ordinator is allocated to and responsible for each client

- highly co-ordinated, intensive service with brief daily handover meetings and weekly clinical review meetings

- extended hours, seven-day-a-week service with capacity to manage crises and have daily contact with clients where needed

- time-unlimited service, with continuity of care.

A meta-analysis of assertive outreach trials concluded that teams that meet these criteria achieve better engagement, reduced hospital admissions, increased independent living and increased user satisfaction (Marshall, cited in DH/CSIP, 2005). In particular, the team approach where the team as a whole manages the caseload was seen as a key feature associated with better outcomes.

However a survey of its members conducted by the NFAO (2005) has identifed continued problems in achieving the model (see also Priebe *et al*, 2003). In particular, dedicated medical input and access to inpatient beds was seen as lacking. The survey also identified continued problems of recruitment and retention and competition for funding among local teams, with teams seldom fully resourced to meet expectations. This mixed picture is also reflected in the 2005 annual autumn review on progress towards implementation of the NSF, in which only 77% of NSF local implementation teams considered their level of assertive outreach provision to be satisfactory.[1]

The NSF implicitly linked assertive outreach with risk management, stating the aim that: 'Assertive outreach is in place for all individuals who may fail to take their prescribed medication and would then be at risk of depression, severe mental illness or suicide; for those who have a tendency to drop out of contact with services; and for those who are not well engaged with services' (Department of Health, 1999). However, despite some concerns about coercion expressed by users of assertive community treatment (eg. Spindel & Nugent, 1999), some have reported the experience as less coercive than provision by CMHTs and more informal and family orientated (see, for example, Killaspy *et al*, 2006). Users appear to value the frequent contact with team members achieved through a team approach.

Priebe *et al* (2005) explored the reasons for both disengagement and re-engagement among African-Caribbean and white British men. Disengagement was associated with three key themes: (i) a desire to be an independent person, (ii) a lack of active participation and poor therapeutic relationship, and (iii) a sense of loss of control due to medication and side effects. With respect to engagement, the key factors were (i) social support and engagement without a focus on medication, (ii) time and commitment from the staff, and (iii) a therapeutic relationship based on a partnership model. A Department of Health/CSIP (2005) research seminar on assertive outreach has suggested that: 'Consideration should be given as to how the successful features of AO working should be extended to other parts of mental healthcare'.

---

[1] See www.mentalhealthstrategies.co.uk

That said, the likelihood of increased community coercion arising from the anticipated amendments to the Mental Health Act mean that assertive outreach practice – indeed, all community team practice – should be underpinned with clear values as set out, for example, in the 10 Essential Shared Capabilities (NIMHE, 2004). These spell out the importance of 'practising ethically: recognising the rights and aspirations of service users and their families, acknowledging power differentials and minimising them whenever possible… [and] positive risk taking: empowering the person to decide the level of risk they are prepared to take with their health and safety.'

Crisis resolution teams

The MHPIG (Department of Health, 2002) made clear that crisis resolution teams are positioned between community-based referrers and inpatient care and should act as a point of assessment and as a gatekeeper to other parts of the mental health system for people in severe distress. They will therefore usually need the capacity to provide immediate home treatment 24 hours a day, seven days a week. Other key features of CRT operation include:

- remaining involved with the service user until the crisis has resolved and they are linked into ongoing care

- where hospitalisation is necessary, being actively involved in discharge planning and providing intensive care at home to enable early discharge

- working to reduce future vulnerability to crisis.

The MHPIG also highlighted the following key principles of care:

- rapid response following referral

- intensive intervention and support in the early stages of the crisis

- active involvement of the service user, family and carers

- an assertive approach to engagement

- time-limited interventions with sufficient flexibility to respond to differing service user needs

- an emphasis on learning from the crisis, with the involvement of the whole social support network.

CRTs have attracted considerable controversy, with some psychiatrists arguing that they are unnecessary in a UK context (Burns *et al*, 2000), on the grounds that improved communications between existing CMHTs, primary care and inpatient units would achieve similarly improved outcomes (Pelosi & Jackson, 2000) and that mental health services already contain and deliver most of their features.

A systematic review of CRTs (Joy *et al*, 2001; updated 2006) reported only a limited impact on hospital admissions, but found home care to be as effective as hospital care when evaluated in terms of numbers of clients lost to contact, deaths and levels of mental distress. However the review also found that outcomes were dependent on effective implementation: in particular, the routing of all referrals to inpatient care through the crisis resolution service. Where this has been achieved, local services report very significant impacts on acute inpatient admissions.

Although the target of 335 teams in place by 2004 was reported to have been met (Appleby, 2004), this does not appear to coincide with the actual staffing capacity required to deliver an effective crisis response. A national survey in 2005 (Onyett *et al*, in preparation) found significantly fewer teams, as many were amalgamating, usually because of cost pressures. Teams reported operating at around 88% of their MHPIG recommended staffing capacity and seeing 59% of the projected target number of clients. This might just mean the original MHPIG guidance needs to be revised and that CRTs should be seeing a smaller and more targeted group in order to achieve maximum local impact. However, team managers in the survey expressed concern over lack of staff to support effective out-of-hours cover and absence of a co-ordinated local response to crises that made full use of the CRT model. Only 68% of teams claimed that they acted as gatekeeper to acute inpatient beds, and only 40% of the team managers reported they were 'fully set up' to meet the requirements of the MHPIG.

Early intervention teams

As stated above, the aim of early intervention teams is to provide a service to people at an early stage of psychosis, in order to avoid long-term illness and dependency. There are 10 guiding principles to the operation of early intervention services (see *Table 1*).

Building on the pioneering work of Birchwood *et al* (1998), randomised controlled trials have found that clients of early intervention teams report reduced readmissions, improvement in symptoms and better quality of life (Nordentoft *et al*, 2002; Craig *et al*, 2004).

The NHS Plan required the establishment of 50 early intervention services, each covering a population of approximately one million people and managing 150 new cases per year, with a total caseload of approximately 450. In order to reap the benefits of effective teamworking, services would need to subdivide into three or four teams with a caseload of 30 to 50 new cases per year and 120 to 150 in total. The state of knowledge on early intervention at that time meant that these targets were highly speculative. Nonetheless, if realised, these figures would translate into between 150 and 200 teams nationally.

Table 1: The 10 guiding principles of early intervention

1	A strategy for early detection and assessment of psychosis is an essential component of early intervention.
2	A key worker should be allocated as soon as possible following referral in order to develop engagement and rapport and to 'stay with' the client and family/friends through the first three years (the 'critical period'), preferably using an assertive outreach model.
3	An assessment plan and assessment of needs should be drawn up that are both comprehensive and collaborative and driven by the needs and preferences of the client and their relatives and friends.
4	The management of acute psychosis should include low dose, preferably atypical antipsychotics and the structured implementation of cognitive therapy.
5	Family and friends should be actively involved in the engagement, assessment, treatment and recovery process.
6	A strategy for relapse prevention and treatment resistance should be implemented.
7	A strategy to facilitate clients' pathways to work and valued occupation should be developed during the critical period.
8	A key responsibility of the service is to ensure basic needs of everyday living – housing, money, practical support – are met.
9	Assessment and treatment of comorbidity (ie. co-occuring drug or alcohol misuse) should be undertaken in conjunction with that for psychosis.
10	A strategy to promote a positive image of people with psychosis needs to be developed locally.

(from www.iris-initiative.org.uk/guidelines.htm)

Early intervention is the area where there has been least progress in implementation according to the 2005 autumn review.[2] Only 77% of LITs were providing some level of service, and only 35% rated provision as being at a level that would meet local need (approximately the same figure as in the autumn review of two years previously). A survey in 2005 found 117 teams of which 86 had funding and 63 were operational (Pinfold *et al*, in press). Only three teams met all 10 features as listed in *Table 1*. Just over half the teams cited lack of funding as limiting development. The

---

[2] See www.mentalhealthstrategies.co.uk

authors concluded that, despite a rapid growth in EI teams, there were marked regional variations in implementation, and many were fragile. Around a third of the population in England was judged to have no local early intervention service.

Taking local team working forward

Evidence to date suggests that, if properly implemented, these three new community team models can achieve demonstrable local improvements in outcome; that the direction set by the NSF and the NHS Plan is positive, but that there is much work still to do (Appleby, 2004). That said, the wider picture is of significant gaps in community team capacity to deliver in line with the MHPIG and the assessed needs of local people. A recurring theme is lack of staff and the associated issue of poor availability of the right range of psychosocial interventions. The Department of Health has recently (at time of writing) launched a national programme to encourage greater access to psychological therapies but the focus is on common mental health problems and maintaining people in employment. While this is a laudable aim, it does not address the existing shortfall of capacity for people who are already receiving secondary mental health services.

The NIMHE New Ways of Working initiative[2] is also working to modernise existing roles within the mental health system, and to introduce new roles of enormous potential benefit to community team working, such as support, time and recovery (STR) workers. However, there remains an overriding imperative to consider more systematically the deployment of human resources at local level to best meet the need of local communities. NIMHE has developed a tool for teams that will help them develop their own workforce plans (the Creating Capable Teams Approach,[3]) but this will only be effective if the functions and objectives of the teams are clear.

Improved integrated working at a local level requires clarity at commissioning level over the respective priorities of primary care trusts and local authorities, and how they come together. Informed by the shared framework offered by the health and social care white paper Our Health, Our Care, Our Say (Department of Health, 2006), these priorities need to be translated into shared eligibility criteria at local level. There are concerns that the development of foundation trusts, with their greater financial autonomy, may undermine this collaborative approach. Rethink (2004) has also highlighted concerns in the voluntary sector that the implicit focus of the new team models on younger people is increasing the risk that older people with longer-term problems become even more vulnerable to loneliness, isolation and a poor quality of life. It will be crucial that the potential of the voluntary and community sector to help achieve local equity of access is fully realised, and guidance to support such flexible local implementation based on need (NIMHE, 2003) already exists.

---

[3] See www.csip.org.uk and http://kc.nimhe.org.uk

We also need stronger leadership and management. We need to find ways of getting team members to identify not only with their immediate team but also with the work of the local mental health service as a whole. Managers need to come together from across teams within a locality to operationalise agreed priorities and functions across agencies. West (2004) advocated that all local teams include in their objectives that they will act in a spirit of co-operation and altruism to other local teams. Community teams have a large role in achieving local person-centred planning that promotes inclusion, equality and the other key outcomes sought by users, but this requires leadership at the level of localities and communities to ensure that these values are evident at whatever point users engage with local services.

The overriding aim is that teams should be designed around the needs of users and the people that support them. Placing users and their supports at the centre of team operation and improvement means that users should have one co-ordinating staff member with whom they feel they can establish a positive working relationship. Effective relationships are a crucial to creating an environment in which users, their social networks and staff can work together to achieve the best outcomes given the prevailing conditions. Equally crucially, services must be able to offer evidence-based psychosocial interventions and access to other key resources, such as benefits advice (for example, by working in partnership with an independent welfare rights agency or organising an outreach advisor service from Jobcentre Plus), and advice and support on employment and access to education and leisure activities and housing (see SCMH, 2004a; 2004b).

Good quality, enduring relationships are required if teams are to respond to an individual's needs and preferences, particularly when working with clients from black and minority communities (see Fuller, 2000; Onyett, 2003). There are undoubted advantages in a team approach in meeting the diversity of needs of users and their supports through access to a range of staff, but it also needs to be recognised that individuals will form stronger relationships with some team members than others.

Last, but not least, community team workers need to stay healthy and motivated themselves. They need access to those things that give meaning to their work, such as direct work with users in contexts where everyone is able to find an effective role (Onyett, 2003). There is also evidence that staff morale is promoted in teams that are specifically designed to be effective and use best practice based on current available research (Carter & West, 1999).

References

Appleby L (2004) *The national service framework – five years on.* London: Department of Health.

Birchwood M, Todd P, Jackson C (1998) Early intervention in psychosis: the critical period hypothesis. *British Journal of Psychiatry* **172** (s33) 53-59.

Burns T (2004) *Community mental health teams.* Oxford: Oxford University Press.

Burns T, Harrison J, Marshall J *et al* (2000) Psychiatric home treatment. *British Medical Journal* **321** 177.

Carter AJ, West MA (1999) Sharing the burden: teamwork in health care settings. In: Payne R, Firth-Cozens J (eds) *Stress in health professionals: psychological and organisational causes and interventions.* Chichester: John Wiley & Sons.

Craig TKJ, Garety P, Power P *et al* (2004) The Lambeth early onset (LEO) team: randomised controlled trial of the effectiveness of specialised care for early psychosis. *British Medical Journal* **329** 1067-1070.

Department of Health (1999) *National service framework for mental health: modern standards and service models.* London: Department of Health.

Department of Health (2000) *NHS Plan: a plan for investment, a plan for reform.* London: HMSO.

Department of Health (2001) *Mental health policy implementation guide.* London: Department of Health.

Department of Health (2002) *Community mental health teams: mental health policy implementation guide.* London: Department of Health.

Department of Health (2006) *Our health, our care, our say: a new direction for community services.* London: Department of Health.

Department of Health/CSIP (2005) *Assertive outreach in mental health in England. Report from a day seminar on research, policy and practice.* London: Department of Health.

Fuller L (2000) Anti-racist practice in mental health assessment. In: Basset T (ed) *Looking to the future: key issues for contemporary mental health services.* Pavilion Publishing/Mental Health Foundation.

Joy CB, Adams CE, Rice K (2001; updated 2006) Crisis intervention for those with severe mental illness. In: *The Cochrane Library*, Issue 4. Oxford: Update Software.

Killaspy H, Bebbington P, Blizard R *et al* (2006) The REACT study: randomised evaluation of assertive community treatment in north London. *British Medical Journal* **332** 815-820.

National Forum for Assertive Outreach (2005) *Annual report 2004-05.* www.nfao.co.uk

NIMHE (2003) *Counting community teams: issues in fidelity and flexibility.* Leeds: NIMHE.

NIMHE (2004) *The ten essential shared capabilities: a framework for the whole mental health workforce.* London: Department of Health.

Nordentoft M, Jeppesen P, Kassow P *et al* (2002) OPUS project: a randomized controlled trial of integrated psychiatric treatment in first episode psychosis – clinical outcome improved. *Schizophrenia Research 2002* **53** 51.

Onyett SR (2003) *Teamworking in mental health.* Basingstoke: Palgrave.

Onyett SR, Heppleston T, Bushnell D (1994) A national survey of community mental health teams. *Journal of Mental Health* **3** 175-194.

Onyett SR, Linde K, Glover G *et al* (in preparation) *A national survey of crisis resolution teams in England.*

Pelosi A, Jackson GA (2000) Home treatment: enigmas and fantasies. *British Medical Journal* **320** 305-309.

Pinfold V, Smith J, Shiers D (in press) Audit of early intervention in psychosis service development in England in 2005. *Psychiatric Bulletin.*

Priebe S, Fakhoury W, Watts J *et al* (2003) Assertive outreach teams in London: models of operation. Pan-London assertive outreach study part 3. *British Journal of Psychiatry* **183** 148-154.

Priebe S, Watts J, Chase M *et al* (2005) Processes of disengagement and engagement in assertive outreach patients: qualitative study. *British Journal of Psychiatry* **187** 438-443.

Rethink (2004) *Lost and found: voices from the forgotten generation.* London: Rethink.

Sainsbury Centre for Mental Health (2004a) *The Supporting People programme and mental health.* Briefing Paper 26. London: SCMH.

Sainsbury Centre for Mental Health (2004b) *Benefits and work for people with mental health problems.* Briefing Paper 27. London: SCMH.

Spindel P, Nugent JA (1999) *The trouble with PACT: questioning the increasing use of assertive community treatment teams in community mental health.* (http://akmhcweb.org/articles/pact.htm)

West MA (2004) *Building a team-based future.* Presentation given at Team Working Today conference. Royal College of Nursing, 15th November.

Chapter 16
Acute inpatient care: its role and the challenges it faces

Paul Lelliott

A psychiatrist retiring today at the age of 65 will have witnessed a total transformation of mental health services within their working lifetime. In the mid-1960s mental health services were located in large psychiatric hospitals and the focus of care was inpatient treatment. Although there would have been outpatient clinics, community services were absent or, at best, embryonic. The locus of mental health care in England has shifted progressively since that time. Large psychiatric hospitals were phased out and replaced by psychiatric services organised around admission beds in district general hospitals. From the 1980s, English mental health care entered a second stage of development with the establishment of an array of dispersed community services. Today, the preferred locus of psychiatric care is the patient's own home. This process was accelerated by publication in 2000 of the NHS Plan, which focused on the further development of specialist community services and set targets for the establishment of assertive outreach and crisis resolution teams (Department of Health, 2000).

The most noticeable marker of these changes has been the great reduction in psychiatric beds. The number of NHS beds in England has fallen to less than one quarter of what it was in the heyday of the asylum.

The role of acute inpatient care

According to the policy implementation guide (Department of Health, 2002) that followed publication of the national service framework for mental health (Department of Health, 1999):

> '... the purpose of an adult acute psychiatric inpatient service is to provide a high standard of humane treatment and care in a safe and therapeutic setting for service users in the most acute and vulnerable stage of their illness. It should be for the benefit of those service users whose circumstances or acute care needs are such that they cannot at that time be treated and supported appropriately at home or in an alternative, less restrictive residential setting. (Department of Health, 2002)

This definition encapsulates one of the principal problems for acute inpatient services: their role is viewed as simply the default option when care in the community has failed. Their active purpose is ill-defined.

Most admissions to acute psychiatric wards are unplanned and happen at a time of crisis; risk to self or others is the most common reason. The staff responsible for providing care to the person once they are in hospital have little or no say about the decision to admit. Furthermore, the purpose of an admission, beyond that of containment and reduction of risk, is often not adequately communicated by those making the decision to those who have to undertake the subsequent care. This lack of communication makes it difficult for ward staff to maintain a positive attitude to patients and good relationships with managers and with other components of the mental healthcare service (Bowers, 2005).

Bowers (2005), following an examination of the research literature, proposed seven reasons for admission and six functions that are provided by ward nurses (*Table 1*).

Table 1: Reasons for admission to, and functions of, an acute psychiatric ward

Reasons for admission to an acute psychiatric ward
■ Dangerousness ■ Assessment ■ Medical treatment ■ Severe mental disorder ■ Self-care deficits ■ Respite for carers ■ Respite for the patient
The functions of an acute psychiatric ward
■ Providing safety for the patient and others ■ Collecting and communicating information about patients ■ Giving and monitoring treatment ■ Tolerating and managing disturbed behaviour ■ Providing personal care ■ Managing an environment where patients can comfortably stay

(Bowers, 2005)

The NSF policy implementation guide emphasises the importance of 'integrating inpatient care within a whole systems approach' (Department of Health, 2002) and, in particular, the need for links with crisis resolution teams and other elements of the acute mental health services.

Challenges for acute inpatient services

Despite the massive reduction in bed numbers, inpatient provision remains the single most costly element of the mental health service and the one that employs the greatest number of staff (Department of Health, 2002). This is unlikely to change. Bed numbers in England have remained fairly static for the past five years and there is growing recognition that they are close to the irreducible minimum (Mental Health Act Commission, 2005).

The Department of Health has acknowledged that, despite their great cost, inpatient services are a neglected part of the mental healthcare system in England (Department of Health, 2002). In many parts of the country, inpatient provision has developed without systematic planning, while management attention has focused on the new community teams (Mental Health Act Commission, 2005; Sainsbury Centre for Mental Health, 2005). If anything, this tendency has been reinforced by the fact that the NHS Plan and national service framework have mandated new types of community services and directed managers' attention to these developments through the NHS performance management system.

The problems for psychiatric admission wards in England were acknowledged by the NSF (Department of Health, 1999) and, seven years after its publication, there is very good evidence that these problems persist (Healthcare Commission, 2005; Marshall *et al*, 2004; Mental Health Act Commission, 2005; Sainsbury Centre for Mental Health, 2005). These problems, and some of the factors that contribute to these, can be summarised as follows.

A change in the case mix of admission wards compromises safety and quality

The reduction in bed numbers has led to a raising of the threshold for admission and the concentration on acute wards of people with more severe problems who pose greater risk to self and others. In particular, a higher proportion of inpatients are now young men detained under the Mental Health Act; many have co-morbid problems of substance misuse (Fitzpatrick *et al*, 2003; Lelliott, 1996; Phillips & Johnson, 2003). As a result, wards are places where adverse events happen frequently. The vast majority – 83% – of mental health patient safety incidents reported on the national reporting and learning system of the National Patient Safety Agency (NPSA) occur in inpatient settings (Scobie *et al*, 2006). *Table 2* is taken from another report prepared for the NPSA, which reviewed the evidence about the frequency of different types of patient safety incidents on acute wards.

Table 2: Relative frequency of patient safety incidents on acute psychiatric wards in England and Wales

	Estimated no. of incidents each year in England & Wales	Estimated no. of admissions per incident[1]	Estimated interval between incidents for an 'average' ward[2]
Aggression/ minor assaults	300,000	0.5	1 day
Absconding	50,000	3	6 days
Sexual harassment/ assault	45,000	4	1 week
Self-harm	25,000	6	12 days
Absconding – does not return	4,500	35	10 weeks
Death by suicide of an inpatient	200	800	4 years
Unnatural death of detained patient	85	1,800	9 years
Homicide by inpatient	1.3	115,000	600 years

(Marshall *et al*, 2004)

[1] For example, an 'average' ward would have one inpatient suicide for every 800 admissions

[2] For example, an 'average' ward would have one inpatient suicide every four years

Many wards have a poor physical environment

The design and layout of many acute psychiatric wards do not support the provision of safe care or create an environment that respects the privacy and dignity of patients. The Healthcare Commission's National Audit of Violence in 2005 reported that many wards failed to meet basic safety standards (Healthcare Commission, 2005); the patient environment action team inspections concluded that 'overall, standards [of cleanliness] were markedly poorer in mental health hospitals compared to acute hospitals'.

There are problems with staffing and staff morale

The Healthcare Commission suggested that one factor explaining the lower standards of cleanliness in mental health hospitals 'may be low morale and poor levels of staffing' (Healthcare Commission, 2005). There are problems in the recruitment of nursing staff to work in inpatient services. This results in extensive use of agency and bank staff and inexperienced nurses being asked to manage wards (Healthcare Commission, 2005). A survey undertaken by the Sainsbury Centre for Mental Health in 2005 found that the vacancy rate for qualified ward nurses was 13% nationally and 22% in London, and that the average ward employed agency and bank nurses for more than 150 hours each week (Sainsbury Centre for Mental Health, 2005).

Wards provide few therapeutic opportunities for patients

Surveys of service users who have been admitted to hospital show that many patients are dissatisfied with the opportunities offered for therapeutic activities (Rethink, 2004; Rose, 2000). Inactivity and boredom characterise life on the ward, with nurses preoccupied with fire-fighting and dealing with paperwork, with little time to provide therapeutic or leisure activities, or even to talk to patients. The absence of things to do is particularly noticeable during the evening and at weekends (Healthcare Commission, 2005).

A national priority

Recent surveys suggest that the challenges that confront acute inpatient services remain, despite the establishment of 'acute care forums' to oversee local policy implementation. This is perhaps not surprising, given that the problems are the result of years of neglect. The government has made some new investment in acute psychiatric wards, and government agencies responsible for setting standards for and regulating English health services have focused on this element of provision. The National Institute for Health and Clinical Excellence (NICE) has published evidence-based clinical practice guidelines about the management of disturbed behaviour in inpatient mental health settings (NICE, 2005); the Healthcare Commission continues to support the National Audit of Violence, and chose acute services as its mental health thematic review in 2006; the National Patient Safety Agency prioritised safer wards for acute psychiatry as its first topic in mental health (Marshall *et al*, 2004).

Alongside this, the Royal College of Psychiatrists, working with the British Psychological Society, the College of Occupational Therapists and the Royal College of Nursing, has established an accreditation system for acute admission wards (Royal College of Psychiatrists, 2006). A comprehensive set of service standards are applied through a process involving both self-review by ward staff and a peer-review visit by staff from other psychiatric units that are participating in the accreditation process. The expectation is that engagement of front-line staff in this systematic approach to quality improvement, with the support of the network of participating wards, will lead to incremental improvements in service quality. The incentive of accreditation will hopefully encourage service managers and commissioners to make resources available to make any specific changes indicated by the review process.

In addition, NIMHE has been supporting initiatives through its acute care programme: notably the recent London Acute Care Collaborative (London Development Centre/Kings Fund, 2006). This initiative, while limited in its scope, has produced encouraging improvements in patient experience on wards, and evidence that small but important changes can be achieved with very modest investment. Perhaps most significantly, it has shown that making staff more available to patients can reduce adverse incidents, so that acute wards are able to provide a place of therapeutic safety for people in crisis.

What remains clear, by the government's own admission (Appleby, 2004), is that acute inpatient services continue to be regarded as a place of last resort, rather than an integral part of the care continuum. As one patient put it in a Rethink (2005) report:

> '... when the crisis hits you're grateful for [inpatient wards] for the first few days, and then you spend the rest of the time trying to get out of the wards because, you see, they achieve nothing.'

It is often argued that what is needed is a greater range of alternative provisions for people in crisis, including short-stay crisis houses (Mental Health Foundation, 2002; Rethink, 2005) and better resourced outreach, crisis resolution and home treatment teams, thereby reducing reliance on hospital admissions and the resulting dislocation of users from their lives, families, communities and social support systems. However, this systemic thinking, which locates the solution to the problem of the quality of acute wards elsewhere, might be part of the problem itself in that, once again, it diverts the attention of service planners. The quality and safety of acute psychiatric wards will not improve unless there is substantial investment of resources and management time in the development of the wards themselves.

References

Appleby L (2004) *The national service framework for mental health – five years on.* London: Department of Health.

Bowers L (2005) Reasons for admission and their implications for the nature of acute inpatient psychiatric nursing. *Journal of Psychiatric and Mental Health Nursing* **12** 231-236.

Department of Health (1999) *National service framework for mental health: modern standards and service models.* London: Department of Health.

Department of Health (2000) *The NHS plan: a plan for investment a plan for reform.* London: The Stationery Office.

Department of Health (2002) *Mental health policy implementation guide: adult acute inpatient care provision.* London: Department of Health.

Fitzpatrick NK, Thomson CJ, Hemingway H *et al* (2003) Acute mental health admissions in inner London: changes in patient characteristics and clinical admission thresholds between 1988 and 1998. *Psychiatric Bulletin* **27** 7-11.

Healthcare Commission (2005) *National audit of violence (2003-2005)*. London: Healthcare Commission.

Lelliott P (1996) Meeting the accommodation needs of the most severely mentally ill people. *Journal of Interprofessional Care* **10** 241-247.

London Development Centre/Kings Fund (2006) *The acute care collaborative*. London: LDC/Kings Fund. (www.londondevelopmentcentre.org.uk/silo/files/458.pdf)

Marshall H, Lelliott P, Hill K (2004) *National Patient Safety Agency safer wards for acute psychiatry: a review of the available evidence*. London: National Patient Safety Agency. (www.npsa.nhs.uk/site/media/documents/1241_SWAP_ResearchReport.pdf)

Mental Health Act Commission (2005) *In place of fear: 11th biennial report 2003-2005*. London: the Stationery Office.

Mental Health Foundation/Sainsbury Centre for Mental Health (2002) *Being there in a crisis: a report of the learning from eight mental health crisis services*. London: Mental Health Foundation/Sainsbury Centre for Mental Health.

NICE (2005) *Violence: the short-term management of disturbed/violent behaviour in in-patient psychiatric settings and emergency departments*. London: National Institute for Health and Clinical Excellence.

Phillips P, Johnson S (2003) Drug and alcohol misuse among in-patients with psychotic illnesses in three inner-London psychiatric units. *Psychiatric Bulletin* **27** 217-220.

Rethink (2004) *Behind closed doors: acute mental health care in the UK*. London: Rethink. (www.rethink.org/research/pdfs/Behind-Closed-Doors-Report.pdf).

Rethink (2005) *Future perfect? outlining an alternative to the pain of psychiatric inpatient care*. London: Rethink.

Rose D (2000) *Users' voices*. London: Sainsbury Centre for Mental Health.

Royal College of Psychiatrists (2006) *Accreditation for acute inpatient mental health services (AIMS)*. London: Royal College of Psychiatrists. (www.rcpsych.ac.uk/crtu/centreforqualityimprovement/aims.aspx)

Sainsbury Centre for Mental Health (2005) *Acute care 2004: a national survey of adult psychiatric wards in England*. London: Sainsbury Centre for Mental Health.

Scobie S, Minghella E, Dale C *et al* (2006) With safety in mind: mental health services and patient safety. *Patient Safety Observatory report 2*. London: NPSA.

Chapter 17

Toxic environments? violence and aggression on acute wards

Geoff Brennan

Acute inpatient environments have, historically, always struggled to balance therapeutic care with containment. The evolution of mental services, as outlined in Paul Lelliott's chapter, has exacerbated this inherent contradiction. Where once the acute psychiatric ward was the fulcrum of psychiatric service provision, it is now intended to be seen as one section of a continuum of care that starts and ends in the community, with a specific role to play in providing safety as well as treatment (Department of Health, 2002). The reality, however, is that the inpatient psychiatric ward is seen as the place of last resort, and is often experienced (by patients and staff) as an extremely unsafe, untherapeutic place to be – truly toxic environments within toxic institutions (Campling *et al*, 2004).

This is the situation reported vividly in numerous surveys over many years (SCMH, 1998; 2005; HASCAS, 2003; King's Fund, 2003; NPSA, 2006). These commonly report over-crowded conditions, difficulties recruiting permanent staff resulting in lack of continuity and high use of bank and agency staff and reduced opportunity for patient contact, poor physical environments, and lack of privacy. A particular issue is endemic violence, threat of violence, aggression and disturbed behaviours, particularly but by no means exclusively affecting the safety of women patients. In the national audit of violence on inpatient acute psychiatric wards 2003-05, conducted by the Royal College of Psychiatrists for the Healthcare Commission (Healthcare Commission, 2005), 78% of nursing staff reported having experienced violence – either personal attack, threats or feeling unsafe – on their ward, and 89% had witnessed another person being attacked. More than one in three (36%) of patients also reported personal experience of violence and aggression. The NPSA report (2006) in particular highlighted risk of sexual assault and even rape – by staff and by other patients.

Indeed, the most recent biennial report from the Mental Health Act Commission (2005) explicitly borrowed its title from Aneurin Bevan's book In Place of Fear, to which it attached a question mark. The MHAC stated:

'… many people with long-term serious mental health problems are not yet secure in the knowledge that the services they will encounter at moments of acute need will be safe, welcoming or even appropriate places for their care and protection.'

But simply recording the facts does not provide an answer to the question why. What is necessary is to unpack the factors that are contributing to these levels of disturbance and threat. These include:

- a reduction in the number of beds available, resulting in high levels of bed occupancy

- no systematic assessment of staff numbers and skills mix necessary to manage wards (Golden, 2004)

- a diversion of resources to establish the new community services (SCMH, 1998)

- disparities in pay and conditions (particularly for nurses) leading to a migration of experienced staff away from the acute sector

- high absenteeism among permanent staff due to high sickness rates, high vacancy levels and training demand, with little provision for covering absence (McKee *et al*, 2006)

- increased numbers of patients detained under the Mental Health Act with high levels of challenging behaviour and complex health needs (Clark & Bowers, 2002; Garcia *et al*, 2005)

- the change in patient profile from predominantly female to predominantly male (Prior & Hayes, 2001)

- an increase in numbers of patients with factors that predispose towards violence, such as substance misuse and forensic histories (Mullen, 2006)

- increased risk monitoring and management, alongside decreased needs assessment and provision of services (HASCAS, 2003).

In essence, there has been a gradual deterioration of wards in terms of physical environment and a leaching away of human and financial resources, alongside an increase in demand and complexity of clinical presentations. The worsening conditions, as we can see from the above, are an understandable, predictable and natural consequence of the combination of these factors – and they can be rectified.

The MHAC biennial report (2005) provides a grim picture of conditions on the average (although by no means all) inpatient unit:

- shabby and ill-kept wards offering bleak and counter-therapeutic environments

- inappropriate patient mix – patients of widely differing ages and diagnoses crammed together in a restricted area

- little personal space on wards and reduced opportunities to go off-ward because of lack of staff or lack of access to outside areas

- bed pressures leading to patients being transferred or moved between wards, or 'hot-bedding' (where patients are sent home on leave to allow another patient to use the bed)

- mixed units, and sometimes inadequately separated female sections

- drug abuse and drug culture

- wards locked to control drug use and trading

- poor arrangements to meet patients' cultural, religious and communication needs

- very little for patients to do in terms of leisure and/or therapeutic activities.

The national audit (Healthcare Commission, 2005) asked patients and their visitors what, in their view, triggered violent incidents on the ward. The five most frequently cited triggers were:

- substance misuse (including alcohol, illegal drugs and withdrawal from their use)

- staff – staffing levels, skills, experience, attitudes (eg. patronising, custodial, interventions used or absence of interventions, interactions with service users)

- space, overcrowding – bed numbers, unit layout, proximity of other people, lack of privacy

- medication and treatment – side effects, compliance, change to medication regime

- frustration – lack of activities, noise levels, missing family and friends, no visitors.

Other common factors including smoking (lack and presence); excessive noise (doors banging, doorbells, people making noise late at night); intimidation by other service users; theft of personal belongings, and temperature.

In the words of one patient, quoted in the Mind Ward Watch survey (2004):

'The whole ward should be demolished and started again. It's unsafe. Drugs are being bought and sold on the ward. Staff do not seem interested in their jobs. Patients are left to wander around with nothing to do (it's a long day) The place smells like an old ashtray. Service users all feel demoralised and get little help from staff.'

Managing the problem

Much attention has been focused on the violence, and short-terms ways to control and prevent individual acts of aggression safely. Little has been done to address the organisational and systemic issues reflected in these reports. The chief response has been the issuing of guidance on the management of violent incidents (NICE, 2005; NIMHE, 2004). For example, guidance issued by NICE addresses solely the 'short-term' (72-hour) management of violent incidents; there is nothing here that seeks to address the factors known from the evidence to provoke and lead to violence, or the development of therapeutic environments. The emphasis is on risk assessment and risk management, on training staff in de-escalation and safe restraint techniques: a commonsense strategy, and undoubtedly beneficial to hard-pressed staff, except that there are serious doubts as to whether it is possible accurately to identify patients who present a high or low risk (NACRO, 1998). Moreover, such an approach risks creating a suffocating atmosphere, defensive practice (itself counter-therapeutic), and a trigger happy attitude to control and restraint: what Kemshall calls 'risk avoidance and the worship of safety' (Kemshall, 2002).

Interim guidance on managing violence issued by NIMHE (2004) (the full guidance has yet to be published at time of going to print) shares the preoccupation of the NICE guidance. Thus, all trusts must have policies on:

- recognition, prevention and de-escalation strategies
- risk assessment and management
- approaches to actual management of aggression and violence
- use of seclusion
- physical care and observation during and post restraint
- basic life support
- health and safety policies
- post-incident support, review and reconciliation
- root cause analysis and sharing lessons learned
- recording, reporting, monitoring and audit (NIMHE, 2004).

All necessary measures, but all essentially defensive – which is hardly surprising when the guidance itself was rushed out in response to the inquiry into the death while being restrained of David (Rocky) Bennett (Norfolk, Suffolk & Cambridge Strategic Health Authority, 2003).

This is not to say the guidance on the practical management of an incident of violence is not necessary, but it should in no way be seen as the answer to the complex issues described above. Indeed, it could be seen as placing an even bigger burden on the ward environment in that it creates a high demand for training (Allen, 2005), when wards are already over-stretched and lack capacity to release staff for training, even if it were being offered.

And when staff are able to access training, NICE itself casts serious doubts over the content and quality of the courses currently available, which are highly variable and still subject to no national standards. Thus wards are in danger of becoming trapped in a vicious cycle of failure.

Is there a silver lining?

All this points to a failure at national, organisation and systemic levels to address the factors that create such conditions on acute inpatient wards, and to provide resources to enable change. That said, there are some shining examples at local and ward level where steps have been taken that have resulted in a reduction in violence and other unwanted behaviours. What is interesting about these initiatives is that the focus is not on the violence and disturbance; rather, these initiatives have sought to improve physical conditions and the therapeutic environment, and thereby to address the trigger factors. All are characterised by measures that make staff more available and accessible to patients, and improvements in the availability and quality of therapeutic interactions and activities. Key among these initiatives are:

- the Tidal Model. This model seeks to develop therapeutic engagement within a person-centred approach, which has been shown to improve patient satisfaction and reduce disturbed behaviours on wards (Gordon *et al*, 2005; Lafferty & Davidson, 2006)

- the Refocusing Model. This model takes the stance that local clinicians have the answers to local problems and seeks to enable them to effect a realistic plan of change within the individual ward environment (Dodds & Bowles, 2001)

- the City Nurse Project. This is a ward-specific intervention based on assisting local clinicians to analyse the problems and bring about changes to their ward (Bowers *et al*, 2006)

- The Acute Solutions project. This is a national initiative led by the Sainsbury Centre for Mental Health that provided outside support to a number of wards to enable them to identify the problems and own and implement the change process (SMCH, 2006)

- the Acute Care Collaborative (London Development Centre, 2006). This is a London-wide project that provided support, training and guidance, and a small amount of money, to enable front-line ward staff to identify key areas of difficulty and introduce specific changes to address them (see over page).

While these projects are often small and localised – although the Tidal Model is being piloted on a larger scale in Scotland – they do have a common message: that change can be achieved by empowering ward staff and local leaders to provide person-centred care. This leads to better engagement with patients and reported improvements in a variety of outcomes, including reduction in violent incidents.

Small changes, big difference

A total of 34 inpatient acute unit teams from across all ten London trusts providing inpatient care took part in the London acute care collaborative. The explicit aim of the initiative was to 'try out small changes to improve services'; the larger, systemic issues (such as ward staffing levels) were deliberately not tackled. The teams agreed a total of 25 standards that they aimed to achieve by the end of the 15-month initiative. The teams were each allocated £5000 so a project lead could spend one day a week working on the initiative, and to cover specific activities of benefit to patients. By the end, improvements had been achieved on 22 of the 25 standards. Five key standards towards which most teams worked were:

- each ward will have a member of the team who takes a lead on dual diagnosis and receives training and follow-up supervision

- all service users will have met with their primary/named nurse to update their assessment and negotiate their care plan within seven days of admission

- all service users will have a minimum of two one-to-one sessions with their named/ primary nurse per week to review their care plan and update their assessment

- specialist substance use/dual diagnosis workers will provide regular inreach service to the ward (minimum monthly) to provide training, advice, treatment and referral

- each service user will be involved in creating their own activity and therapy programme that will be recorded in their care plan and will include evening and weekend activities.

Three of the most successful and popular changes implemented by the wards were:

- protected engagement time, when the staff office was closed and the ward shut down to all phone calls, paperwork, visitors and other professionals, so staff could engage directly with service users – whether one-to-one or group work, games and activities, escorted leave or meal time supervision

- targeted dual diagnosis training – resulting in a reported change in staff attitudes to one where they are now more prepared to see substance use as part of their job, rather than referring on to specialist substance use teams

- provision for activities – these included staff ensuring all patients got up in the morning and providing a full range of activities to motivate them, outings, patients cooking their own breakfasts, and women's and men's groups.

The report concludes:

'This is a timely reminder of the potential that exists within our acute wards, if only it can be supported and encouraged… We would like to think that, with senior level commitment, making such time and resources available should be within the power of all trusts providing acute inpatient psychiatric care and would lead to measurable benefits' (London Development Centre, 2006).

There are other such initiatives running in wards across the country, often supported by the acute care forums set up under the mental health policy implementation guide for adult acute inpatient care provision (Department of Health, 2002), with input from the NIHME regional development centres. In many cases these changes have taken place in the face of extreme difficulties, many of which arise from the systemic and organisational issues outlined above. As the Sainsbury Centre observes in its summary of the results from Acute Solutions:

> 'Our experience of working with four trusts over the past three years is that progress can be made given the right support for staff and involvement of service users, families, managers, community teams and services. Other parts of the mental health system need to understand and respect the part that acute inpatient care plays... If acute inpatient care is to change fundamentally we need greater clarity about its role and function.' (SCMH, 2006)

Added to this, there also needs to be a reversal of the asset stripping that has leached resources out of acute inpatient services, and the recognition that these services are as important as any other in the whole system of care. These improvements achieved at local level cannot be sustained if problems at organisational levels are not addressed.

References

Allen D (2005) Nice guidance but timing is off. *Mental Health Practice* 8 (7) 14-15.

Bowers L, Brennan G, Flood C *et al* (2006) Preliminary outcomes of a trial to reduce conflict and containment on acute psychiatric wards: City Nurses. *Journal of Psychiatric and Mental Health Nursing* 13 165-172.

Campling P, Davies S, Farquharson G (eds) (2004) *From toxic institutions to therapeutic environments*. London: Gaskell.

Clark N, Bowers L (2002) Psychiatric nursing and compulsory psychiatric care. *Journal of Advanced Nursing* 31 (2) 389-394.

Department of Health (2002) *Mental health policy implementation guide: adult acute inpatient care provision*. London: Department of Health.

Dodds P, Bowles N (2001) Dismantling formal observation and refocusing nursing activity in acute inpatient psychiatry: a case study. *Journal of Mental Health and Psychiatric Nursing* 8 (2) 183-188.

Garcia I, Kennnett C, Quraishi M *et al* (2005) *Acute care 2004*. London: Sainsbury Centre for Mental Health.

Golden M (2004) Workforce planning: is there a right way? *Mental Health Practice* 7 (10) 33-35.

Gordon W, Morton T, Brooks G (2005) Launching the Tidal Model: evaluating the evidence. *Journal of Psychiatric and Mental Health Nursing* **12** 703-712.

Healthcare Commission (2005) *The national audit of violence (2003-2005)*. London: Healthcare Commission.

Health and Social Care Advisory Service (2003) *Improving the quality of psychiatric inpatient care in London (IQPIL)*. London: Health and Social Care Advisory Service.

Kemshall H (2002) *Risk, social policy and welfare*. Buckingham: Open University Press.

King's Fund (2003) *London's state of mind: King's Fund inquiry*. London: King's Fund.

Lafferty S, Davidson R (2006) Putting the person first. *Mental Health Today* (March) 31-33.

London Development Centre/King's Fund (2006) *Acute care collaborative: trying out small changes to improve services*. London: London Development Centre/King's Fund. (www.londondevelopmentcentre.org)

Mental Health Act Commission (2005) *In place of fear? 11th biennial report 2003-05*. Nottingham: MHAC.

McKee P, Harrison A, Smith G (2006) Nursing establishments within acute inpatient mental health units: the need for clarity. *Mental Health Practice* **9** (8) 18-21.

Mind (2004) *Ward watch*. London: Mind.

Mullen PE (2006) Schizophrenia and violence: from correlations to preventative strategies. *Advances in Psychiatric Treatment* **12** 239-248.

NACRO (1998) *Risk and rights: mentally disturbed offenders and public protection: a report by NACRO's mental health advisory committee*. London: NACRO.

NICE (2005) *Violence: the short-term management of disturbed/violent behaviour in in-patient psychiatric settings and emergency departments*. London: NICE.

NIMHE (2004) *Developing positive practice to support the safe and therapeutic management of aggression and violence in mental health in-patient settings*. Leeds: NIMHE.

NPSA (2006) *With safety in mind: mental health services and patient safety*. Patient Safety Observatory report 2. London: NPSA.

Norfolk, Suffolk and Cambridgeshire Strategic Health Authority (2003) *Independent inquiry into the death of David Bennett*. Norfolk: Cambridgeshire Strategic Health Authority.

Prior P, Hayes B (2001) Changing places: men replace women in mental health beds in Britain. *Social Policy and Administration* **35** 397-410.

Sainsbury Centre for Mental Health (1998) *Acute problems: a survey of the quality of care in acute psychiatric wards*. London: Sainsbury Centre for Mental Health.

Sainsbury Centre for Mental Health (2005) *Acute care 2004: a national survey of adult psychiatric wards in England*. London: Sainsbury Centre for Mental Health.

Sainsbury Centre for Mental Health (2006) *The search for acute solutions*. London: Sainsbury Centre for Mental Health.

Chapter 18
Dual diagnosis: working with people with mental health and substance use problems

Iain Ryrie

Substance use among people with mental health problems can present significant challenges for the individuals themselves, for their families and for those who provide care. Historically in the UK, substance use and mental health services have evolved separately; few services are equipped to manage both conditions. However, innovative service models have been reported in the literature, and a dual diagnosis good practice guide has been published by the Department of Health (2002). This chapter builds on these developments and begins with an overview of the nature and extent of substance use among people with mental health problems, including possible reasons for use and their associated health implications. The chapter then turns to matters of policy before considering approaches to treatment and care.

Overview of dual diagnosis

Although the term dual diagnosis may seem straightforward, the range of people categorised in this way is extremely diverse (Kipping, 2004). Take, for example, a university undergraduate who uses drugs recreationally and suffers a panic attack the morning after a drug-fuelled Saturday night party. Or a man who experiences an acute psychotic episode and turns to alcohol to quieten the persecutory voices that taunt him. In both cases it is possible, if not necessarily desirable, to apply the term dual diagnosis. To unravel this complexity the Department of Health (2002) presents two intersecting axes: one that represents the severity of mental health problems and one representing the severity of substance use (See *Figure 1* over page).

Figure 1: The scope of mental health and substance use problems

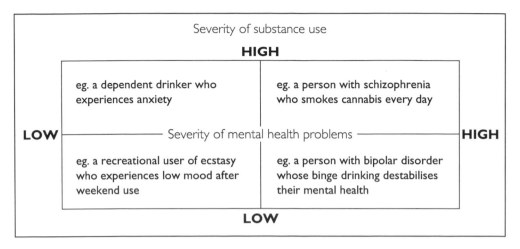

It follows from *Figure 1* that a range of causal factors may be involved in the development of different types of dual diagnosis. They have been summarised as follows:

- a primary psychiatric illness can precipitate or lead to problematic substance use
- substance use can worsen or alter the course of a psychiatric illness
- intoxication and/or substance dependence can lead to psychological symptoms
- substance misuse and/or withdrawal can precipitate or lead to psychiatric symptoms or illness. (Crome, 1999, Mueser *et al*, 2003)

Government policy and the literature to date have primarily focused on those individuals in the right hand quadrants of *Figure 1*: that is, those people with severe mental health problems who also use substances. Research data suggest that these people are at significantly greater risk of developing a substance use problem than the general population (Regier *et al*, 1990, Menezes *et al*, 1996). It is thought that between 30% and 50% of people with severe mental health problems also use substances, and the Department of Health advises that substance use should be considered usual rather than exceptional among this group (Department of Health, 2002). The gravity of this situation is highlighted by the consequences of substance use for many of these individuals. Higher rates of homelessness, suicidal behaviour, violence and HIV infection have been reported, together with increased use of institutional services, a worsening of psychiatric symptoms and poor adherence to medication (Menezes *et al*, 1996; Banerjee *et al*, 2002; Department of Health, 2002).

It's also important to understand why such people continue to use substances, despite their consequences. Phillips and Johnson (2001), in a review of the literature, found that people with severe mental health problems use substances to cope with low or sluggish mood states, anxiety and sleeplessness. Others suggest that substances are used to manage hallucinations and disturbing thoughts, or to cope with the side effects of psychiatric medications (Mueser *et al*, 2003). It's also understandable that a socially marginalised group that experiences disadvantage and stigma may from time to time seek escape through the use of substances. These possible reasons for substance use emphasise the value individuals can place on the activity. In turn, health and social care staff must take account of these reasons and temper their approach accordingly. For example, in the immediate term at least, it may not be realistic to insist on abstinence.

Policy

While different strands of national policy have historically focused on either substance use or mental health problems, it is now understood that 'joined up' policy is required if the needs of people with a dual diagnosis are to be comprehensively met. The dual diagnosis good practice guide (Department of Health, 2002) introduces an emerging policy framework to achieve these ends based on 'mainstreaming' the care of people with severe mental health and substance use problems in mental health services, which are now required to take lead responsibility for their care. While the term 'mainstreaming' implies the routine acceptance and management of individuals with a dual diagnosis by mental health services, it does not represent a lessening of the input from the substance use sector. Joining up policy in this way necessitates closer working between the two, which means:

■ substance use services providing specialist support, consultancy and training to mental health services to support their care of clients with severe mental health problems

■ mental health services offering similar packages of support to substance use services so that they can provide comprehensive care to people with less severe mental health problems. (Department of Health, 2002).

These reciprocal support mechanisms are primarily focused on individuals with severe mental health or substance use problems. However, from *Figure 1* it is clear that other individuals may encounter dual diagnosis problems without necessarily coming to the attention of specialist services. Furthermore, current drug misuse and dependence guidelines (Department of Health, 1999a) emphasise a key role for GPs in the management of substance use problems. There is then a need for joined up policy that incorporates primary care. The National Service Framework for Mental Health (Department of Health, 1999b) emphasises this point and advises that primary care assessments of individuals with mental health problems should always consider the potential for substance use. Similarly, the assessment of individuals with severe substance use problems should include consideration of their mental health status (Department of Health, 1999a). However, assessments are only really useful if adequate treatment and care responses are available. Thus, primary care staff should have a working knowledge of how to access specialist services, and the reciprocal support mechanisms recommended for 'mainstreaming' in specialist mental health services should also be available to primary care services.

Local implementation teams across mental health services (LITs) and drug action teams across substance use services (DATs) have been established to support the implementation of these policies. There are then strategies, teams with responsibility for their implementation, and practice guidelines for bringing together mental health and substance use services. However, there is another policy strand that significantly affects the likelihood of success. The commissioning or purchasing of services must also follow these policy developments. In recent years services have increasingly been commissioned by primary care trusts. Thus, future success will depend in part on LITs and DATs co-ordinating and communicating service development plans. Equally, it is necessary for primary care commissioners to develop their knowledge of this complex field (Department of Health, 2002).

The national director for mental health Louis Appleby, in his five-year review of the national service framework for mental health (Appleby, 2004), describes the impact of these initiatives as 'modest'. Despite evidence of effective partnerships between DATs and LITs, by 2004 only 17% of LITs had produced a dual diagnosis strategy and the Department of Health has requested further improvements in joint planning and commissioning.

Treatment and care

Different ways of providing services have been reported in the literature, including serial, parallel and integrated models (Department of Health, 2002). The former implies the treatment of one problem or condition before receiving treatment for the other. Since substance use and mental health problems can interact with one another (see *Figure 1*) this type of approach is problematic. Both conditions need to be attended to simultaneously.

The parallel model allows for this possibility as each condition is treated at the same time but by different services. Closer working between substance use and mental health services may make this a viable operating model. However these partnerships are intended to enable 'mainstreaming', rather than the treatment of the different conditions by different services, even if it is at the same time.

The integrated model originates from the US, where specialist hybrid teams with both mental health and substance use expertise have been established to support individuals with a dual diagnosis (Drake *et al*, 2001). However the UK's health and social care infrastructure is different to that in the US, and the Department of Health believes integrated treatment can be better achieved here through its 'mainstreaming' policy – by lodging integrated care in mental health services with liaison and support from the substance use sector – as described above. There is potential for variations on this theme, as described in the good practice guide: one example is augmenting mental health teams with a specialist substance use worker (Department of Health, 2002).

Framework for delivery

Detailed descriptions of treatment and care are beyond the scope of this chapter. However, there are some general principles that can be usefully outlined here. Since substance use behaviours often follow a long-term course it can be difficult to know how and when to help. Insisting on abstinence may not always be realistic: put simply, the individual has to be ready to change. Prochaska and DiClemente (1986) suggest the following seven stages that people go through in relation to behavioural change:

- pre-contemplation – behaviour not seen as a problem
- contemplation – some acceptance of problem
- decision – to address the problem
- active change – steps taken to change
- maintenance – work to maintain gains
- relapse – return to pre-change behaviour, or
- change fully adopted.

The full adoption of change may require several attempts. The framework indicates that if someone is at the pre-contemplation stage it may be more appropriate to help them develop an awareness of any problems associated with their substance use than to try to negotiate their stopping. That may come later when the individual is able to make the decision for themselves.

Another useful framework relates to the stages of treatment and was originally reported by Osher and Kofoed (1989):

- engagement – developing a trusting relationship
- persuasion – exploring problems, weighing up pros and cons, educating
- active treatment – changing substance use behaviours
- relapse prevention – support to maintain change.

Once again, the nature of substance use behaviours is such that progression through these stages of treatment may take months, but is more likely to take years. It's necessary for health and social care staff to take a long-term view, and for continuity of care to be fostered over time. The 'stages of change' and 'stages of treatment' frameworks provide a guide to the types of interventions that should be offered at any point in time. We need in the first instance to listen to the individual service user. What are they telling us about their needs and their readiness to change? With an understanding of their perspective and an appreciation of the different 'stages' of change, we will be better placed to offer appropriate, timely and ultimately useful interventions.

References

Appleby L (2004) *The national service framework for mental health – five years on*. London: Department of Health.

Banerjee S, Clancy C, Crome I (2002) *Co-existing problems of mental disorder and substance misuse (dual diagnosis): an information manual*. London: Royal College of Psychiatrists Research Unit.

Crome I (1999) Substance misuse and psychiatric co-morbidity: towards improved service provision. *Drugs: Education, Prevention and Policy* **6** 151-174.

Department of Health (1999a) *The national service framework for mental health: modern standards and service models*. London: Department of Health.

Department of Health (1999b) *Drug misuse and dependence: guidelines on clinical management*. London: The Stationery Office.

Department of Health (2002) *Dual diagnosis good practice guide*. London: Department of Health.

Drake R, Essock S, Shaner A *et al* (2001) Implementing dual diagnosis services for clients with severe mental illness. *Psychiatric Services* **52** 469-476.

Kipping C (2004) The person who misuses drugs or alcohol. In: Norman I, Ryrie I (eds) *The art and science of mental health nursing*. Maidenhead: Open University Press.

Menezes P, Johnson S, Thornicroft G *et al* (1996) Drug and alcohol problems among individuals with severe mental illnesses in South London. *British Journal of Psychiatry* **168** 612-619.

Mueser K, Noordsy D, Drake R *et al* (2003) *Integrated treatment for dual disorders: a guide to effective practice*. New York: Guilford Press.

Osher K, Kofoed L (1989) Treatment of patients with psychiatric and psychoactive substance abuse disorders. *Hospital and Community Psychiatry* **40** 1025-1030.

Phillips P, Johnson S (2001) How does drug and alcohol misuse develop among people with psychotic illness? a literature review. *Social Psychiatry and Psychiatric Epidemiology* **36** 269-276.

Prochaska J, DiClemente C (1986) Toward a comprehensive model of change. In: Miller W, Heather N (eds) *Treating addictive behaviours: processes of change*. New York: Plenum.

Regier D, Farmer M, Rae D *et al* (1990) Comorbidity of mental disorders with alcohol and other drug abuse. *Journal of the American Medical Association* **264** 2511-2518.

Chapter 19
Commissioning mental health services: towards social inclusion

David Seward

At its most basic level, commissioning is the process whereby the mental health needs of a local community are assessed, and the assessment then translated into a strategic plan for the provision of mental health services to meet those needs. The plan states who provides the services, where they are provided, and at what standard of quality. These services are then 'purchased' from provider organisations – NHS mental health trusts, the voluntary sector, or the independent sector. Commissioning is a continuous process. Service provision should be subject to continual review in terms of quality and performance, and in the light of changes in local health needs.

At the time of writing primary care trusts (PCTs) in England, and health boards in Scotland, Northern Ireland and Wales, are the bodies with statutory responsibility for commissioning all health services for their local populations, working with their partner local authorities, who have the same function for social care services.

Consequently, commissioning can be seen as simply a mechanism for allocating funding to mental health services and professionals so they can direct their attentions where they are most useful and most needed. However, it also provides a safeguard to ensure that NHS services are indeed directed towards patient need, and not steered by the particular interests and concerns of the provider organisation and the health professionals working in it.

Therefore, while the process is relatively straightforward, the mechanism is more complex. The basic structure – that of separating the commissioner (the PCT) from the provider (the mental health trust or other provider of services) – was established in 1989, in the policy paper Working for Patients (Department of Health, 1989). This deliberately created a competitive environment on the basis that an 'internal NHS market' would drive up quality of care by creating a purchasing body that had no stake in the provider function and could therefore take a clearer view of local need. In theory, it could also introduce greater choice and drive down costs of health service provision, by encouraging competition between provider bodies.

In addition, commissioning was always meant to be done in partnership with local stakeholders, including statutory and non-statutory providers and service users and carers. It was recognised that those best placed to understand local need and locally appropriate service responses were the people providing the services, because they were in direct contact with the local community. As a result, local health and social care communities have established various joint planning groups that bring all stakeholders together to support statutory commissioning bodies with their work. This is broadly the framework today, midway through 2006, but – as ever – the situation is in constant flux and shortly to change yet again.

However, while mental health service provision may have changed radically in the last ten years, improvement in both effectiveness and efficiency of service provision has generally lagged behind other parts of the NHS (SCMH, 2005). More importantly, while we have seen considerable change with the move from institutional to community based care, an even greater change is yet to come. Current government policy is to break down the 'asylum walls' that still separate people with long-term mental health problems from the communities in which they live (SEU, 2004). The goal now is social inclusion, equality of opportunity and access, and mainstreaming service provision. Wherever possible, people with mental health problems will be supported back into work (or other meaningful activity), into independent living and into using the public services to which we are all equally entitled. More broadly, the aim for the population at large, in line with public health policy in general, is to prevent mental ill health occurring in the first place, by tackling the main factors known to impact on individual and community mental well-being (NIMHE, 2005; Department of Health, 2004a; 2006).

If social inclusion and community mental well-being is to become a meaningful reality for all, how, where and by whom mental health services are to be provided requires radical review. Mental health and the factors that impact on it cross every government departmental boundary. Service provision to address mental health needs therefore involves a very wide array of stakeholders – health, social services, education, employment, housing, transport and more – and, of course, a pooling and significant redistribution of resources among the various partner organisations.

The perception is that mental health commissioning in its current form has not been up to the task. In which case, it is unlikely to be able to push forward a social inclusion agenda (Department of Health, 2005a).

Structures and systems

Another challenge for current commissioning arrangements is the perceived prescriptive nature of the immediate policy framework.

The national service framework for mental health (Department of Health, 1999) and accompanying policy and implementation guidance (Department of Health, 2001), coupled with an emerging best practice evidence base and a whole industry developing around targets and performance management, means that traditional tasks of commissioning are losing their relevance. What mental health services are supposed to provide is set out very clearly in the framework and implementation guidance; there is very little room for deviation, and there are annual, national targets to ensure commissioners and providers comply. Local commissioning can therefore be seen as having little relevance when there is such clarity about the models of care to be provided, and centralised targets dictate priorities at local level.

In addition to the mental health national service framework, the organisations that commission and provide mental health services are changing. PCTs have been merged into a smaller number of much larger organisations, supposedly in order to provide better strategic oversight. It was argued that PCTs were too small to employ sufficient specialist mental health commissioners to achieve the level of change and improvement required in mental health services. Some PCTs attempted to address this by giving one of their number, within a local consortium, lead responsibility for mental health issues. However this created problems in that the lead PCT often lacked authority to commission on behalf of the others within the grouping. The problem with the larger PCTs is that they risk becoming too distanced from the communities they serve.

Partly to redress this, a further development is the roll out of practice-based commissioning (Department of Health, 2004b; 2005c). This brings micro-commissioning decisions back under the influence of individual GP surgeries and local communities. Essentially, clusters of GP surgeries working with other local stakeholders will receive an amount from the PCT budget to commission local mental health services specifically for their practice populations' needs. The idea is that this will complement the improved strategic planning achieved by the larger PCTs.

At the same time, foundation trusts are being introduced, and it appears clear that they are intended to become the norm. Foundation trust status gives mental health trusts greater control over their own finances and the services they provide: they can seek contracts from any commissioning body, not just their local PCT (Department of Health, 2005b). Their greater independence as quasi-autonomous service providers is potentially underpinned by payment by results (PbR) (Department of Health, 2004b; 2005c). Traditionally, PCTs have purchased mental health services from provider organisations through block contracts, either on a year-by-year basis or a rolling, three-year cycle. Some contracts also have service level agreements attached that specify in more detail what these services will provide and the quality outcomes expected. PbR (at time of writing it is yet to be rolled out to include mental health services) differs radically from this; instead trusts are paid for each item of service, operation or course of treatment they perform. However it may not be well suited to a condition such as mental ill health, where episodes can be of any length, outcomes are uncertain and unpredictable, recovery and maintenance are subject to so many factors outside the control of the health service, and where relapse and fluctuation of illness are so common.

There are a number of commissioning models that might accommodate the challenges presented by mental health. These have been usefully summarised by the NHS Confederation with Rethink (2005). One option is the HMO model, whereby PCTs and or local practices contract a specialist commissioner to buy service elements from a range of statutory and non-statutory specialist and general health care providers, within a fixed programme budget. Another alternative is the long term conditions model, which uses a fixed tariff payment mechanism based on predicted costs of 'year of life with condition' to cover. This builds on practice-based commissioning in that practices would buy packages of services from statutory and independent providers, who in turn may subcontract elements of provision to other organisations. This approach actively incentivises early intervention and promotion of recovery, as these would lead to reduced dependency over the long-term. Both have advantages in that they keep the provider–commissioner split and permit choice around individual need. However, there are still the problems of expertise, and hence power, predominately lying with the provider organisations, as well as the increased bureaucracy of managing the payment system.

Which way forward?

It is unclear what impact practice based commissioning will have and how successfully it will work alongside strategic PCT planning. Commissioning-type tasks, such as need assessments and monitoring quality of service delivery, will undoubtedly be done at various levels and by many different organisations, who will continue to work from different perspectives and with different priorities. Arguably, this scenario will replicate the existing arrangements that have produced disappointing results precisely because the multiple stakeholders in the mental health arena operate in an unco-ordinated way, and in some cases work against each other. What, therefore, might unite these activities and set an agenda to which they could all work?

The basic model for secondary mental health care services is relatively clear, set within by the national service framework. However it is also possible to see a common thread running through current health and social care policy that sets a new and rather more challenging agenda for mental health and mental well-being: that of social inclusion, choice and recovery. Simply procuring a mental health service that is compliant with policy and implementation guidance will not in itself address these new priorities. Improving standards of practice, addressing clinical governance and responding better to patient satisfaction issues all help advance the quality of service and undoubtedly form an important part of the work for those with commissioning responsibilities, in whichever part of the system they sit. However, commissioning really needs to prepare current services and wider stakeholders for a very different future, and a very different way of meeting mental health needs.

This shift in perspective is typified in the report, The National Service Framework for Mental Health – Five Years On (Appleby, 2004), which moves the focus on from the 1999 NSF to address social exclusion, improving responsiveness to ethnic minority communities and increasing access to alternative interventions in primary care, such as psychological therapies and general health care for long-term mental disorders. This community-building agenda for mental health is further emphasised in the Social Exclusion Unit report on mental health (SEU, 2004), which sets out a 27-point action plan for tackling stigma and discrimination and for improving access to employment, and to social, educational and community opportunities. This emphasis on social inclusion opportunities is underpinned by a new, optimistic philosophical perspective that sees mental ill health as something from which people can recover, and that expects the mental health practitioner to respond positively to the aspirations of service users and carers (NIMHE, 2001). This is a significant departure from traditional assumptions that regarded severe mental illness as permanently disabling, with consequent implications for service design and delivery.

The implications for mental health service organisation and delivery are significant. It requires a much closer level of integration between health and social care and primary and secondary care. More importantly, it envisages specialist mental health, generic health and the whole gamut of social care services, including providers of transport, housing, employment, education, benefits and pensions, prioritising mental well-being and the creation of healthy communities. It also sees new partnerships between the statutory, voluntary and independent sector, and these being extended to connect with the commercial sector, and service user-run social enterprise.

What commissioning might look like in the future is, at this point, difficult to predict. However the direction of travel for mental health services is beginning to take shape. In a report setting out their vision of mental health services in 2015, the Local Government Association, the NHS Confederation and the Sainsbury Centre for Mental Health (SCMH *et al*, 2006) predict that the focus of all public services – health, social services, education, employment, housing, transport and more – will be on mental well-being, and that specialist mental health services will be more integrated into generic health, social and community care services.

One possible vehicle for responding to this changing policy framework is the social forum model (NHS Confederation/Rethink, 2005). This involves the creation of local partnership boards that bring together the strategic planning functions and relevant funding streams of all statutory health and social care, employment and benefits bodies within local authority areas.

Such a partnership would enable a much more radical approach to delivering opportunity and choice by overcoming the interface issues that have to date prevented a seamless and coherent approach to realising the recovery and social inclusion agendas. Partner organisations and agencies would contribute funds to a shared pot from which a broad-based mental well-being service could be commissioned from a wide variety of providers. While there are questions as to the sustainability and practical application of this model, the emerging policy framework for mental health services make it a strong option for the future.

Any real change to mental health requires a radical deconstruction of traditional institutional services, treatment options, workforce parameters and cultural perspectives (Hurford & Seward, 2005). In the end, simple economics and changing workforce demographics may be the catalyst for making this change happen. There is now increasing awareness of what the real costs of a comprehensive mental health system are, and the likely shortfall in what we as a nation can afford. This, coupled with the evidence of the economic and social cost to society of mental illness, makes a compelling case for reform (SCMH, 2003). In the short term, practice-based commissioning supported by improved strategic planning at PCT level is likely to be the way forward. However something more radical will be required in the long-term if we are to achieve social inclusion and promote community well-being.

References

Appleby L (2004) *The national service framework for mental health – five years on.* London: Department of Health.

Department of Health (1989) *Working for patients.* London: The Stationery Office.

Department of Health (1999) *National service framework for mental health: modern standards and service models.* London: Department of Health.

Department of Health (2001) *Mental health policy and implementation guidance.* London: Department of Health.

Department of Health (2004a) *Choosing health: making healthier choices easier.* London: the Stationery Office.

Department of Health (2004b) *NHS improvement plan: putting people at the heart of public services.* London: Department of Health.

Department of Health (2005a) *Commissioning a patient-led NHS.* London: Department of Health.

Department of Health (2005b) *A short guide to NHS foundation trusts.* London: Department of Health.

Department of Health (2005c) *Creating a patient led NHS: delivering the NHS improvement plan.* London: Department of Health.

Department of Health (2006) *Our health, our care, our say.* London: the Stationery Office.

Hurford H, Seward D (2005) Commissioning and opportunities for re-engineering. *Primary Care Mental Health* **3** (4) 275-278.

NHS Confederation/Rethink (2005) Mental health – the commissioning challenge. *Consultation* **21** (September).

NIMHE (2001) *The journey to recovery.* Leeds: NIMHE.

NIMHE (2005) Making it possible: improving mental health and well-being in England. Leeds: NIMHE/CSIP.

Sainsbury Centre for Mental Health (2003) *The economic and social cost of mental illness.* London: SCMH.

Sainsbury Centre for Mental Health (2005) *Beyond the water tower.* London: SCMH.

Sainsbury Centre for Mental Health/Local Government Association/NHS Confederation (2006) *The future of mental health: a vision for 2015.* London: SCMH/LGA.

Social Exclusion Unit (2004) *Mental health and social exclusion.* London: Office of the Deputy Prime Minister.